To Kim,

[signature]

10/15/06

What You Need To Know
About U.S. Health Care

YOUR HEALTH
MATTERS

Gregory Dattilo, CEBS
& David Racer

Alethos Press LLC.

i

ALETHOS PRESS LLC
PO Box 600160
St. Paul, MN 55106

Your Health Matters: What You Need to Know About U.S. Health Care
ISBN 0-9777534-0-9

Printed in the U.S.A. by Bethany Press International, Bloomington, MN

Cover Design by Risdall Advertising Agency, New Brighton, MN, and Bethany Press International

http://www.yourhealthmattersbook.com

10 9 8 7 6 5 4 3 2 1

TABLE OF CONTENTS

Authors' Introductions

Gregory Dattilo

For more than 30 years I have worked in one small corner of the United States health care system. It is a complex system that employs tens of millions of people. It is a system always undergoing transition.

I have witnessed a long string of medical miracles that resulted from the incredible creativity of men and women who have been motivated to extend human life, and to reduce pain and suffering. My journey has been exciting, fulfilling, and rewarding.

As I have visited my elderly mother, I often reflect on the medical miracles afforded our senior citizens: new hips and knees, motorized carts, drugs to spare them from pain or extend their lives. In many foreign countries, where they do not enjoy the financial successes we Americans take for granted, many seniors die from lack of care or suffer excruciating pain; because their country's health care budget cannot support their needs.

I watch children, and I know that not so long ago, many would never have survived childbirth. I know that in many foreign countries, there is very little effort to save the lives of the tiniest babies. They do not save them because the costs could not justify their health care treatment.

I have seen employees of my clients recover from devastating diseases, to return to work and live productive lives. I have, likewise, seen a good number of human health tragedies, but most often, these people receive high quality medical treatment, even when their chance of survival is slim.

During these 30 years, I have had the pleasure of helping hundreds of employers and their employees find health insurance to meet their needs. I have watched the U.S. health insurance system grow from an affordable and effective program, to one that is becoming too expensive for some of my clients. From a system that relied on patient responsibility, I now see a system that tries to do everything for everyone at others' expense.

I have worked around these trends, managing health benefits as best I can, always grateful for the good that our system delivers to my clients. Lately, however, I have begun to grow concerned as I witnessed the dual predicament of rising insurance costs, and a concerted effort by powerful interests to shift the responsibility for health care away from private markets and to the federal and state governments.

This book needed to be written so that Americans can be informed about the health care choices that they must make in the years to come. David and I commend it to you, because your health matters.

THANKS TO SOME VERY SPECIAL PEOPLE

I wish to express my thanks to many people who made this book possible.

First, my co-author, David Racer. More than 15 years ago I heard David on the radio as I drove to an appointment. At that time, he hosted a talk radio show, The Dave Racer Show on a Twin Cities radio station. As I heard him talk about health care issues, I was amazed; he actually talked with authority and knowledge. So we had lunch, and that developed into a working relationship, and then a friendship. David's ability to take complex issues and condense them into understandable writing is truly remarkable. His story-telling melded perfectly with the technical and experiential knowledge I brought to the partnership, and it added humor and color to the book. Both of us enjoyed researching the various subjects, and our follow-on discussions brought many issues out of the shadows, so that we could bring them to you in clear light.

Secondly, David and I want to thank Jo McClaine, our St. Louis, Missouri friend, who did such a great job proofreading the boook (okay, I made that misteak on porpose).

Thirdly, I want to thank my employees. They had to pick up and complete many tasks that I normally do, and keep me on schedule and focused on business, even while my mind was on the next chapter that David and I planned to write.

Next, I want to thank my children – Gregory II, Ivy, and Grant – for sharing me with the book. We love to do things together, but during the 14 months it took to put this book together, that time was often sacrificed.

To my wife Joan, I offer unending thanks and love for her encouragement in so many ways, but mostly, for the time she sacrificed that we usually spent together. And thanks for letting David and I spread out our work on the kitchen table, even while you tried to get things done around the house.

I would be remiss without thanking the dozens of employers who form my client base. What I have learned from them and their employees during the past 30 years gave me the insights and a good deal of the inspiration I needed to make this book come to life.

DAVID RACER

Gregory called me during the late fall of 2004 and said he wanted to write a book about the United States health care system. He knew it would be a big project and hoped I had the time and interest to help him. I jumped at the chance.

Health care is the issue that first brought Gregory and me together during the early 1990s. The two of us created quite a stir at the Minnesota legislature with the materials we released about health care, and other business issues, so the adventure of doing a book on health care immediately appealed to me.

Neither of us knew that it would consume 14 months of our lives. Of course we knew that the system was wide-ranging, decentralized, and chaotic. Sometimes, trying to pull it all together so that the public could understand what we wrote felt a bit like herding cats. Yet, it has been an immensely satisfying task, and we seemed a perfect fit to get it done.

Gregory is extremely knowledgeable about the insurance side of the health care equation, and he is a keen observer of people, government, and economics. His analytical mind, combined with specific knowledge and the determination to know details, balanced my sometimes-greater desire to "make the narrative sing." Gregory loves the United States, free markets, family, all the good things about our country, and has a profound concern that we make good choices about our future. That is why he invested so much of himself, his fortune, his time, into this book.

I, too, want to thank my wife Rosanne for tolerating yet another writing venture. She really is a great companion for a writer, willing to sit and listen to my repeated ruminations about the subject material, and rant about the frustrations of writing a book. She encouraged me constantly to keep on, stay up late, get up early, do whatever it took to complete this book.

One of the difficulties of writing a knowledgeable book about health care is that the system is never static. It is constantly changing. This makes presentation of facts more difficult because, inevitably, the statistics are always out of date. It takes those responsible to assemble the data 12-24 months or more to verify and release the new numbers. Even at that, they often revise one year's calculations months or years after they are released. So, the data is always outdated.

As we assembled this book, new data was constantly being released. Most of our statistics deal with the year ending 2003, but many are drawn from other years. This difficulty did not significantly change the substance of this book nor its conclusions.

DEDICATION

This book is written in honor of my father, George Dattilo, the gentlest man I ever knew. Dad spoke very few words. He never tried to tell me how to live. When he did speak, his words carried special meaning.

One phrase that dad repeated often, and that has stuck with me is, "When you believe you're right, don't back down." It is in that spirit, and the motivation I gained from dad's advice, that I offer this book.

Gregory Dattilo

Many people have greatly influenced the way I think about economic and social policy. My ninth grade civics teacher James Phillips, Ph.D.; the fellows at The Foundation for Economic Education; Alan Keyes, Ph.D.; Dr. Richard L. Reece, M.D.; and my good friend Dr. Harold D. Kletschka, M.D.; a list far too long for this meager space. I dedicate my work on this book to all of these, plus the two most humble people I have ever known. They were the ones who allowed me the freedom to continue writing, and encouraged me to persevere – my parents, David and Alice Racer.

David Racer

CHAPTER 1
WHY THIS BOOK?

We think you ought to know the whole story of the United States health care system. For far too long, the news has been dominated by myths and misconceptions, and truth has been buried.

The purpose of any health care system is to protect and preserve human life, to reduce or eliminate pain and suffering, and to improve health. Nothing else really matters if life itself is threatened by illness or injury. And if we live with chronic pain and suffering, every part of our life is affected constantly.

The U.S. health care system is the result of our willingness to spend whatever it takes to preclude pain and delay death.

There is no other industry in which Americans have so much at stake than our health care system. As a result, almost every aspect of U.S. commerce and government touches the health care system in some way, either adding to or taking away from our drive toward the best care in the world.

The U.S. health care system is complex and confusing. In this book, we make it understandable by breaking it down into each of its parts – patients, providers, and pay-ers. We show how each part fits together to provide health care for us all.

Everyone concerned about his or her health, or that of a loved one, should read this book. The truth is that your individual choices, and those made by others you know, ultimately will decide our health care future. This book will help you understand the health care system so that you can make informed, wise, and good choices, and better under-stand the public debate about U.S. health care.

You will be surprised as you read about the U.S. health care "crisis," infant mortality, life expectancy, the unin-sured, the cost of prescription drugs, and the health care issues faced by other nations.

You will be amazed by the untold truths that are some-times purposefully hidden from you.

You will see how the government has, in the past, responded to each health care "crisis." This will help you judge for yourself the direction in which some health care reformers think it should go now.

You will discover the true factors that drive up the cost of health care, and how you can control and influence health care spending. Most of all, you will be able to let political and health care leaders know that you want them to improve the system, expand access, control costs, while making sure not to stifle it or cause it to break down.

The authors' goals are to:

1) expose health care myths;
2) eliminate your misconceptions about health care;
3) allow you to impact today's decisions about tomorrow's health care system;

4) support that which will continue to improve the quality of your health care; and

5) demonstrate how you can access even more health care services, without decreasing quality.

We offer this book to you for a single reason: Your health matters. And unlike some other modern nations, in the United States you still get to choose the future of your own health care.

CHAPTER 2
HEALTH CARE
ALWAYS MATTERED

Since the first settlers walked ashore at Jamestown, Virginia, we have had a health care system. That first system worked poorly, since nearly everyone died within three years.

The fact is that wherever people live, some form of health care system has to exist – even though it might be barbaric and risky, or professional and relatively safe.

In our early days, a little boiled water served as sterilization. A shot of whiskey combined with biting down on a stick served as the anesthetic. Infections were often cured by sawing off an arm or leg. People endured this agony because they loved life so much or feared death more.

By visiting historic United States cemeteries, you gain a simple knowledge of how long people lived during each era. The geographic, climatic, social, and economic conditions where people lived and died are reflected in the ages of those who lie in their cemeteries.

In the cemetery behind Christ's Church in Philadelphia, you will find the headstones of many of those who signed our Declaration of Independence and Constitution.

You will also find the tombs of their infants and older children. This is true of all cemeteries from the United States' earliest days, where headstones bear the names of young children, snatched by death in an epidemic – or taken by simple sicknesses like tonsillitis.

By the turn of the twentieth century, things had not improved much. "Overall, life expectancy in 1900 for the states that provided information was a mere 47.3 years."[1]

Life expectancy is a result of many factors. Among those that figured into the difficult lives of the earliest Americans were:

- high infant mortality – many babies died at birth or shortly after;
- high maternal mortality – giving birth carried a high risk of the mother's death;
- nearly non-existent formal health care – self-care was the norm.

From a point where professional health care barely existed, we have built an incredibly successful health care system. But why? What drove us to demand that our health care system must do everything it could to protect us from the inevitable?

SURVIVAL

Each human is driven by the need to survive. Entire government and social structures are established for that single purpose: that we might live. Health care is a direct link to survival, and it is the most easily identified evidence of our drive to maintain human life.

"I'm bleeding. Get me to the doctor!" "I'm having chest pains. Call 9-1-1!" At the scene of an auto accident, emer-

---

1. Amanda Gardner, "Americans Living Longer, Experts cite better treatments for heart disease," *HealthScoutNews Reporter*, March 14, 2003, http:www.hon.ch/News/HSN/512229.html

gency workers call in an air ambulance to shave a few minutes off the rush to the hospital, making the difference between life and death.

When death threatens, everything else becomes secondary. The drive for survival takes first place – always. It is King of the Hill, the Primary Objective.

As death threatens, extreme emotions surface. Not many emotions exceed these felt by parents at the birth of a child. Still, even that joy fades compared to the raw emotions of parents who have experienced a child's death. Health care sits at the center of these two extremes – birth and death.

The health care system, then, touches the most extreme emotions of all of us, with the real potential at any moment in time to provide inexpressible joy and hope, or unbearable sorrow and pain.

Each morning, most of us wake up assuming we will enjoy good health and safety, while others feel fortunate to have just one more day, though they may dread the pain they must endure. In the back of our minds, we know that the U.S. health care system is ready to care for us if our health is threatened in any way.

SOME Q & A

Question: What do parents fear the most?

Answer: Losing a child, or even using the words, "a child died." In fact, so painful is the subject that today's parents say, "losing a child" rather than "a child died," or "my child died."

Our great-grandparents, living a century ago without the medical miracles that we take for granted, often dealt with a child's death. All they could really do about it was to have more children. They hoped for a long life for each of their offspring, but lived in the reality that their children could die from any number of minor illnesses or simple accidents. The United States' early health care system offered them very few options to save the life of a sick child.

Question: What is the second greatest fear of most parents?

Answer: Losing a spouse: that is, having his or her spouse die. Here again, we prefer to talk of "loss" rather than death.

For most of us, death is the ultimate fear producer. Death is, frankly, the Great Motivator that keeps the health care system in business.

Think of the conversations between our great-grandparents as they talked about the idea of having another child.

"Well," Grandpa asked, "do you think we should go through it again? Will we lose another baby at birth?" He looked Grandma in the eye and added, "Or maybe this time, I'll lose you. I wish there was a way to see if you are at risk from having another child."

Unfortunately, for Grandpa and Grandma, the only "way" was to give birth to another child and hope for the best. Parents a generation later, however, refused to accept the unknown. They demanded that the health care system give them an informed diagnosis, and that it reduce the rate of infant mortality. They were willing to spend more money to protect unborn children and mothers.

Question: What is our most common fear about our own health?

Answer: Having to live with uncontrollable chronic pain and suffering.

The United States' primitive health care system had very few options to relieve pain. One of the most common procedures was amputation. Losing a limb meant shedding a deadly infection, but the procedure itself carried a high risk of death, not to mention excruciating pain. Herbs and roots served as salves to treat wounds. Sometimes, chicken soup really was the only available treatment.

Doctors and medical researchers searched for better, safer, and more successful ways to eliminate pain and suffering, or make life more comfortable for those with chronic pain. Americans used their creative enterprise and a lot of money, and became the world's leader in medical innovation during the twentieth century.

U.S. health care, from 1607, when the first settlers landed at Jamestown, to our day 400 years later, became a system that constantly chases improvement. But during most of that time, until the 1930s, improvements were slow and medical care remained crude.

UNITED STATES CULTURE AND ECONOMY PRODUCED MEDICAL PROGRESS

Question: What invisible forces drove people to invest their lives and fortunes in the advancement of the quality and quantity of the U.S. health care system? How were those forces different from other nations?

Answer: The same love and emotion that drove our great-grandparents drives us today. It causes us to protect the lives of our loved ones, and to treat and relieve pain and suffering.

But why did it take so long for the breakthroughs that led to the modern practice of medicine?

There are several major forces that, over time, contributed to our unique and great success. These forces

9

flourished in our free society, as we cherished individual choice and promoted the sacred nature of human life. Controlled societies with strong, central governments struggled and lagged behind the United States precisely because they lacked these core values.

◆ Culture of Work: The idea that people, regardless of class distinctions, are responsible to earn their own way and provide for their own family.

◆ Ownership: The opportunity to profit from innovation.

◆ Discretionary Income: Enough money to purchase improved services.

◆ Technology: Research producing "miracles" upon which new discoveries are built.

EARNING OUR WAY

U.S. health care evolved rapidly during the twentieth century. It could not have done so unless Americans believed in the value of individual work and earning one's own way. For a limited time, that was not true of our first settlers, when some people felt that they had special privileges that isolated them from work.

Most of the first colonists died within three years of landing at Jamestown, Virginia in 1607. The problems presented by the diseased-riddled place where they chose to settle would have been tough enough, but their lives were made even more miserable by several stubborn aristocrats. Those aristocrats thought that others should do the work, and that they were entitled to position and leisure at the expense of the lower class. While the farmers, craftsmen, and artisans went to work, the aristocrats sat back, expecting others to provide their needs. Everyone suffered.

After the "starving winter" of 1609, of the 500 settlers who had come to the place, only 60 still survived. The fact that the aristocrats refused to work had placed an added burden on everyone that contributed to this needless death.

Captain John Smith's edict, "He that will not work shall not eat," became the byword of those 60 survivors. The hundreds of thousands of colonists who followed later put into practice this same idea, and it still dominates U.S. society, government, and economy: we believe that people ought to work to provide for their own needs. This makes us different from most other nations.

We especially expect new immigrants, even illegals, to find gainful employment. The United States is the country to which people from across the world flock, because we offer them hope. That hope stems from the chance to find work that pays far more than they could earn anywhere else in the world. We attract people who are willing to work, we attract the smartest and the most creative people, because it is here that they can gain benefit from their work. Today, "Many primary care doctor training slots are being filled by internationally trained doctors."[2] The United States offers them rewards unheard of in their native lands.

Americans heartily endorse a culture of work, and the world knows it.

During the heyday of the Soviet Union, a radio interviewer asked a farm expert, "What is the difference between a Soviet and a U.S. farmer?"

"The Soviet farmer goes home at the end of the work day. The U.S. farmer stays on his tractor, working into the wee hours of the morning with his headlights on, until the crop is harvested. After all, he owns the farm."

2. Richard L. Reece, M.D., "For Young Doctors, It's Not Marcus Welby's Practice," 2005,1.

As a result of our culture of work, we have reaped a bountiful harvest of benefits still uncommon to those in societies where the economy is controlled by central governments. One of those benefits is the high quality and sheer number of health care options we take for granted.

GAINS FROM OWNERSHIP

Question: Alongside the culture of work, what other factors have distinguished us since the United States' founding?

Answer: Ownership is a major factor.

The U.S. economy and many of our constitutional freedoms find their root in the idea of private ownership. We can own real estate, businesses, stocks, bonds, and money, and use this as we choose. In recent decades, even communist and socialist nations have begun to understand this, and have moved slowly toward an ownership society.

Ownership allows us to purchase what we want, when we want it. Those who have money left over after purchasing basic needs are driven to invest in new products and services that generate greater personal wealth. This is called capitalism: investing capital – money – to create more wealth.

Since the continuous drive to improve health care stems from an unquenchable desire to live longer, free from pain and suffering, capitalism finds a way to deliver this to us. Imagine the investor who searches for a place to put his or her money and finds a chance to own a piece of the next major breakthrough in medical devices: The risks are great, but the rewards are even greater. The investor realizes two great benefits: increased personal wealth and a hope that when he or she needs health care, it will be there waiting to ward off pain, suffering, and death.

12

In the United States, people choose to invest their own money as they see fit or take jobs that they find attractive. There is no government gatekeeper telling them that they must sacrifice ownership for the greater good, or take the job that central planners have chosen for them.

Those other countries that have government gatekeepers spend less of their gross domestic product (GDP)[3] on health care than we do – perhaps eight percent compared to our 15 percent – but they have no choice. Their people are less wealthy and refuse to pay higher taxes to get more health care. Yet, they still want what Americans have: nearly unlimited health care choices and no waiting lines. We, on the other hand, work harder and longer, to earn and spend more to gain better health care.

Money flees to the United States in much the same way as job-hungry immigrants come searching for work. Foreign citizens who have managed to become wealthy invest their money in the U.S. because they have nearly unlimited choices, precisely because no government gatekeeper tells them where they must invest their funds. They know that they will gain more by investing in U.S. industry and commerce, than by giving up their ownership to a central government.

Ownership, then, has provided tens of billions of dollars to be invested in ideas to extend life and reduce suffering. It is the fuel that has driven medical advancements during the last 60 years. This did not happen by accident.

America's continuous march toward greater economic success was made possible because of the choices set in motion by our country's founders. They believed in a free market economy – free enterprise – where individuals, not governments, decide how to invest and spend their own

---

3. *The Concise Encyclopedia of Economics* states, "Gross domestic product (GDP), the official measure of total output of goods and services in the U.S. economy, represents the capstone and grand summary of the world's best system of economic statistics."

money. These free choices, when matched by American ingenuity and hard work, created the wealth that became available to fund medical miracles.

Hard work and capitalism, however, needed two more elements to bring about our medical revolution. Increased discretionary income and technological advances gave the capital somewhere to go.

FRUIT OF HARD WORK IS DISCRETIONARY INCOME

Question: What about U.S. workers? Aren't their choices one of the keys to the improvements in the health care system?

Answer: Absolutely. Workers and their families are the ones who purchase health care services. Their willingness to spend money for their own health care tells providers they need to continuously improve the system.

The astounding success of the U.S. economy has meant that many of us are able to afford to purchase goods and services in excess of that which is required to meet our basic needs. We enjoy the fruit of discretionary income.

The definition of basic needs differs from person to person. Some see a used compact car as a transportation need, while others "need" an SUV and a luxury automobile – in the United States, it is their choice, based on what they can afford. As we use it here, basic needs are food, shelter, clothing, and transportation.

In many other nations, citizens have little or no discretionary income; most of their money goes for basic needs or to pay high taxes that provide a wide array of government services, like health care. We in the United States have far more health care choices compared to other nations because we enjoy greater discretionary spending. In many foreign nations, while common citizens must seek

14

health care from a government-gatekeeper system, those with discretionary income fly to the U.S. to see medical specialists.

The U.S. free market economic system has grown stronger each decade, fueled by citizens choosing how to spend their own money. We believe that each of us is capable of making our own spending choices, rather than having a central government choose for us.

Capitalists and consumers, making their own freewill choices, built the U.S. economy. Our high-quality health care system is the result of a free market that provides us with nearly unlimited choices about how to spend our discretionary income. We use some of that money to buy health insurance to reduce our personal risk, and some of it to purchase optional and alternative health care services and products.

Americans had very little discretionary income until the 1970s, and then, consumers began spending. They bought a second car, a TV for the bedroom, a home entertainment center, or took vacations. Millions of people put money into retirement plans. During this same time, employers began asking their workers to use a small portion of their discretionary income to pay a piece of their own health insurance cost, paid by payroll deductions. Most people went along, because the cost was low.

Most employees only paid attention to their take-home pay, so payroll deductions were a painless way to offset some of the costs of health care. Those 1970s-era payroll deductions of $5, $10, or $25, taken from each employee, created a huge pool of money when they were combined with the insurance premiums collected from tens of thousands of employers.

Congress liked the payroll deduction system so well that it decided to use it to fund a major expansion of the health care system. In 1965, Congress ordered that taxes should be deducted from your check to pay for Medicare and Medicaid (see chapters eight and nine). When these new taxes were combined with that of all working people, it amounted to tens of billions of dollars. The federal government spent those dollars in the health care system. As a result of the government spending your money in this way, artificially stimulating the health care economy, it helped trigger the continuous increases in the cost of individual health care.

Government spending combined with private health insurance to make available a huge pool of money to purchase an increased number of health care services. At the same time, more working people had enough discretionary income to afford services that may not have been covered by insurance. They chose optional health care services and products because they had the money to do so.

So, discretionary income has been a major factor that allowed us to progress from self-care to professional care.

Tens of billions of dollars invested by capitalists combined with hundreds of billions more spent by Americans choosing to purchase better health care, infused the system with what it needed to push for more medical breakthroughs. This vast amount of money made it possible for technological advances that would astound Great-Grandpa and Grandma.

U.S. TECHNOLOGY LEADS THE WORLD

Technology is the result of a process where today's researchers build on yesterday's progress for tomorrow's breakthroughs. This process drives innovation and an unending search for more successful ways to provide your health care. When fueled by the billions of dollars invested by capitalists and consumers, technology results in incredible health care breakthroughs.

During the 1950s, members of the U.S. armed forces used the world's first "portable" computer. Powerful trucks pulled the three semi-trailers of equipment required to make that "portable" work. One trailer carried the tape drives; one carried the generators; the third carried the controls. Today's handheld computers are faster, more powerful and have memories that far exceed that 1950s computer dinosaur. Computer power doubles every 15-18 months because of technological improvements.

Competition drove these advancements. Inventors working out of their garages or basements, and the entrepreneurs who funded them, raced to create new products that would astound the world, and make them a fortune. Small start-up companies, fueled by venture capitalists, took new products to the market, and made their owners wealthy. Big corporations and their stockholders, too, had to compete to grow new products, so that their employees and investors could be rewarded. The world benefited from this keen competition from a vast array of ever-increasing health care choices.

The cold war competition between the United States and the Soviet Union, as well as the race to the moon, further drove the pace of technological change during the 1950s and 1960s. Scientists and inventors created completely new kinds of metals that withstood heat and corrosion, and were far stronger than common steel. Medical researchers found incredible applications for plastics, and combined them with these new metals to create devices used to help people walk, breathe, and even exist. They used the breakthroughs in computer technology to devise entire new ways of practicing medicine.

Today's heart attack victim can often return home from

the hospital in 24 hours. Technology allows a surgeon to insert a miniature camera through a tiny incision in a leg, and then guide it up toward the heart, and then insert a drug-coated stent into an artery to restore blood flow – and save a life. During the 1970s, this type of heart surgery required splitting open a chest, stopping the heart, and performing intricate cardiovascular surgery. The recovery meant a six-week hospital stay. Today, inserting a stent in an artery means an overnight hospital stay. Not only are the patient's risks lower, the relative costs of repairing a damaged heart have declined.

Diagnostic tests, made available through new computer technology, allow a surgeon to spot problems and design medical strategies at an early disease stage. You lie still on a table as a scanner probes your body and a computer analyzes the findings. The doctor reads the results, and knows what to do, all without dangerous, expensive, and invasive exploratory surgery. These diagnostic machines cost millions of dollars, money that comes from capitalists and your discretionary spending.

Other machines can analyze a drop of blood to diagnose many varieties of problems, even years before they become life-threatening. Scanners and MRIs spot cancer in its earliest stages, providing hope for a cure and for longer life.

U.S. medical researchers use technology to reduce pain and suffering, and to increase mobility. New hips and knees allow people to walk without pain. Prosthetic devices replace amputated limbs, allowing people to pursue jobs and careers. Motorized wheelchairs, pain controllers that administer drugs; the list seems endless.

Unfortunately for most citizens living in foreign countries, their government-delivered health care systems restrict the amount of money spent on medical research, or their high taxes discourage it. So, the United States leads the world in technological advances, and foreign citizens with their gatekeeper health care systems play catch-up. Money from private investors makes it possible for new technology to take root. The money we spend on health care shows these investors and researchers that it is worth it for them to take the financial risk to create new technology.

Underneath it all, though, is the strongest of all motivations – the mutual self-interest we have in extending our lives, and to reduce our own pain and suffering.

THE TEST THAT GREAT-GRANDPA WANTED IS NOW COMMON

Just a century ago, our grandparents worried that their newborn baby or the mother would die during childbirth. They wished for a way to see if there were such a risk before the baby was born. Modern technology has created that "way." Doctors view a full-color, four-dimensional ultrasound image to examine a baby while it still swims in its mother's womb. Then they can devise a strategy to save that baby's life if they see it has problems.

Tiny babies achieve healthy lives today. For babies who are carried to term, less than three out of a thousand will die at birth.[4] Grandma would have loved those odds.

Life expectancy in the United States is now nearly 78 years for newborn babies, and increasing all the time. People are living longer and staying active for many more years than their parents did.

Physical pain and suffering has been made tolerable or eliminated for millions of Americans.

---

4. "National Vital Statistics Report, Vol 50, No 12," U.S. Census Bureau, Aug. 28, 2002, 1.

The quality and quantity of U.S. health care has grown dramatically in the last 60 years. There is every indication that medical researchers will continue their relentless pursuit of even better health care for all of us, unless we make the wrong choices.

The United States is unique among the nations of the world in nearly every aspect of life and commerce, and so is our health care system. We are a wealthy people willing to spend whatever it takes to prevent pain and suffering, and extend human life.

Question, with no answer: When will we have spent enough money to preserve and extend life, or to reduce suffering to zero?

CHAPTER 3
IS U.S. HEALTH
CARE TERMINAL?

Question: U.S. health care is in a time of crisis, isn't it? And if we don't fix it soon, you won't be able to get even basic health care. In fact, isn't it true that millions already are denied health care?

Seemingly every day there is a news story to remind you of the grave condition of the health care system. Given these grim reminders, surely the U.S. health care system must be about the worst in the world, except for some third world nations (and maybe we're not so far ahead of them).

The U.S. infant mortality rate ranks forty-third in the world among modern nations at 6.88 deaths per 1,000 live births, while Singapore has the lowest rate at 2.27 per 1,000.[1] Other reports state that U.S. life expectancy ranks seventeenth in the world, while others rank us even worse.

Recent reports state that more than 45 million U.S. residents are uninsured, and the number grows worse each day. Furthermore, media tells us that 18,000 uninsured

---

1. "Table 010: Infant Mort Rates & Life Exp at Birth, by Sex," U.S. Census Bureau International Data Base – 2002.

people needlessly die each year. How can this be in the world's richest nation?

Employers have been hit by enormous increases in health care insurance premiums, and they have asked employees to pay more of their own costs. Some employers no longer offer health insurance benefits, while others offer policies with high deductibles. Shouldn't government require employers to provide health insurance, and force them to pay the entire premium?

Why does health care cost so much, anyway?

Doctors make too much money, right? And isn't it true that hospitals and clinics charge too much, while their executives are paid enormous salaries?

Aren't lawyers getting rich as they bring frivolous lawsuits that sap tens of millions of dollars out of doctors and hospitals?

Isn't it true that Big Drugs (the pharmaceutical companies) only care about profits, and that their profit margins are obscene? What about all those drug and medical device failures? It sounds as though Big Drugs cause more harm than good. And why must U.S. residents order drugs from Canada to save money?

"I put Grandma in a private nursing home," you say, "and they charged us more than $5,000 a month for basic care.[2] It is outrageous!" Yet, isn't it true that nursing home operators complain they cannot continue in business without charging even more?

Then there are those people using government-paid entitlement programs. Do they get too much free care? Do they get too little free care? Do they get any care? Should you even care?

Is the health care system broken beyond repair, as these

---

2. MetLife General News: Press release, April 2002, shows an average daily rate of $168, or $61,320 annually.

media reports imply, and if not, why is it that we constantly hear all this glum news?

WHY ALL THE NEGATIVE NEWS?

Thousands of people are paid to study and design reforms for the health care system, while others earn their living writing and reporting on health care. Some reformers love our health care system, while others think it needs to be replaced. Many of these reformers urge the United States to adopt a health care system managed and funded by the federal government.

Health care reformers from all sides of the debate hear the nearly constant complaints about the system. Doctors complain about reimbursement rates, regulations, paperwork, medical malpractice insurance, and worst of all, insurance clerks telling them how to practice medicine. Insurance companies complain about "utilization," that is, doctors prescribing too many tests, drugs, and surgeries, and patients demanding too many services. Employers and employees complain about premium increases, and higher deductibles and co-payments. Drug and medical device companies complain about over-zealous government regulators who complicate the process of bringing new products to market, and they really dislike state attorneys general and plaintiff's attorneys who sue them. All these complaints offer the media a buffet of negativity on which to graze.

One group of reformers in particular seize on the negative reports, using them to demand a complete overhaul of health care. They prefer a single-payer, government-gatekeeper system.

Some politicians use the negativity for their personal political gain. They focus on, and then parrot back the system's problems, and hold themselves out as the problem-solvers. They say that health care is an entitlement – the government owes it to you – implying that if you elect them, they will ensure that you will have access to afford-able health care; even free health care. They link long life to your vote.

When you hear about the United States' high infant mortality rate or that our life expectancy is less than some other countries, Big Government reformers seize on this to prove that we need change. They also cite our rate of unin-sureds as a moral failure. We discuss these in chapters 11, 12 and13).

Pharmaceuticals are expensive, and some people have trouble affording them. The reformers seldom explain how drug prices are determined. Instead, they want the federal government to purchase them for you, or they recommend importing them from Canada or Europe (see chapter10).

The media loves controversy and negative news. Sel-dom do they feature stories about the tens of thousands of Americans who live with a perfectly functioning defibrilla-tor (an implanted device that shocks your heart if it stops beating). They prefer stories about a handful of defibrilla-tor failures that contributed to people's deaths.

Media reports, and the claims of Big Government advocates and the politicians they favor, almost always lack context. Their 10-second sound bites and press confer-ences pass as truth. Yes, there is a good reason why many in the United States believe we are suffering a health care crisis. They never hear anything but doom and gloom.

DOES THE U.S. SUFFER FROM A HEALTH CARE CRISIS?

The fact is that the U.S. does not have a health care cri-sis. The United States is the world's leader in cutting-edge medical care. The U.S. system provides outstanding health care.

Health *care* is not our problem. Health *cost* is the issue. Consider France during August 2003. "[As]Europe sweltered under a heat wave...more than 15,000 people died in France, dwarfing the number of deaths in neighboring countries."[3] Now, that is a health care crisis!

It is true that the U.S. health care system is expensive. As a nation, we spend about 15.3 percent of our Gross Domestic Product on health care.[4] How does our 15.3 percent of GDP compare to other modern nations?

Country	% of GDP Spent on Health Care
Germany	11.1%
France	10.1%
Canada	9.9%
Japan	7.9%
United Kingdom	7.7%

Source[5]

Obviously, we spend a great deal more of our GDP on health care than other modern countries do, and our $11.1 trillion GDP dwarfs theirs. So our total spending on health care, likewise, dwarfs that of other countries.

If cost is the issue, "Why can't the government order health care providers to reduce their prices?" you might ask. This is the way prices are set in health care systems run by government gatekeepers, like in Canada. If we adopted the Canadian system, perhaps we could spend just 9.9 percent of our GDP on health care as they do.

Many small-government reformers believe that the government created most of the health care cost problems

---

3. *Bulletin of the World Health Organization*, March, 2004, 82(3), page 232.

4. This 15.3 percent calculation is for 2003, and is cited in numerous places. Our source is the Center for Medicare and Medicaid Services news release for January 11, 2005.

5. "Total expenditure on health - % of gross domestic product," OECD, 2003, http://www.oecd.org/dataoecd/44/18/35044277.xls

through over-regulation, taxation, and the scores of mandates it has forced onto insurance companies and medical providers. They believe that if government would quit meddling so much and let the free market do its job, prices would come down and the quality of care would increase even more.

Some well-meaning people go so far as to say that people should pay all of their own health care costs. If they did, they reason, prices would have to fall.

Between the extreme views, government-run health care and people paying for all their own health care, there are as many ideas about how to control health care costs as there are species of fish in the ocean. People on the extremes may not agree how to control health care costs, but they do agree with you and us about this: Costs are high and are going higher.

So what are the factors that influence the cost of health care?

PERSONAL CHOICE IN THE HEALTH CARE ECONOMY

In at least three significant ways health care pricing is different from all other products and services that we purchase. 1) When you are injured or very ill, health care is not an optional purchase. 2) Most health care costs are paid by someone else. 3) We expect the health care system to spend whatever it takes to help us regain our health, treat our suffering, or extend our life until all hope is lost.

Unlike health care purchasing, in our free market system the price we pay for something is determined by supply and demand. The purchase price adjusts itself to what we are willing to pay for it. If we want to buy more of something, suppliers tend to produce more of it, and if they do not, the price will rise.

We usually pay more for scarce items. As we continue to purchase something, competitors step in and offer it for less money – the supply increases and the price drops.

When the government grants patent or copyright protection to something, its price tends to be higher, because there is no competition among suppliers. The price will rise to the highest level that people are willing to pay. When a popular item no longer has patent or copyright protection, competitors step in and offer it at a lower price. This is the pricing cycle of almost everything in a free market system.

For a free market to work best, consumers must have maximum freedom to choose from among a number of options. Price will respond to consumer demands.

In many foreign countries, the government owns major industries and productive property. It may even own everything. In those types of centrally controlled economies, the government decides which products and services to offer and in what quantities. Consumers have few or no choices. This is called a command economy. The price of something is determined by government-appointed committees, ministries, secretariats, academics, and scientists – ultimately, politicians. In these economies, price is not the real issue; availability is the issue. Everyone can afford the product, but almost no one can get it because there are always supply shortages.

People who live under a command economy do not have to worry about the price of health care; they just hope it will care for them when they get sick. People who live under a free market health care economy seldom worry about availability; they are often concerned about increasing costs. In the command economy, if a pipe bursts in your government-owned apartment building, you can be sure that the repairman will show up within a few days, or weeks – but the service will be free. In a free market, dozens of plumbers are ready to show up at your door within minutes, as long as you can pay the bill.

YOUR LEAKY PIPES

Suppose you come home one day and, looking up, you notice wet spots on your kitchen ceiling. You determine it comes from leaky water pipes in the upstairs bathroom. If you do not take care of the problem soon, your house could suffer major damage.

Your first call is to your insurance agent. He informs you that since the pipes are old and the damage is caused by normal wear and tear, insurance will not pay to fix them. He offers to send out an insurance adjuster to explain this, and says that repainting the kitchen ceiling would be covered. Your $500 deductible means, of course, that you would end up paying to paint the ceiling anyway, so you thank your agent and make other plans.

You call a friend who recommends a plumber, and you find another in the Yellow Pages. Plumber one says you really should replace all the pipes in your home at a cost of $18,000. Plumber two says that you can get by with just doing the upstairs bathroom and the pipes near the water heater in the basement, for $5,000. You choose the cheaper option, but must secure a short term bank loan to pay for the repairs. You pay the plumber $2,500 the day he starts, and the rest on the day he finishes. The whole process takes a week, and you hope the other plumber wasn't right about the other pipes in the house.

When you notice a puddle near the water heater a few days later, the plumber comes back and fixes it at no extra cost.

As it concerns your body, while you are feeling good,

you make many health care choices that affect your costs. You make choices about doctors, hospitals, and clinics. You choose the frequency of care and to a great extent, the type of care. You choose a diet, how many hours you sleep, and whether to exercise.

If you choose to have a physical, you learn that you are healthy or that your "pipes" need fixing. You can choose, with your doctor's advice and agreement, whether to take certain drugs, have surgery, visit specialists – and you can do your homework on which specialists to choose. If you have a high deductible insurance policy, you may choose generic or over-the-counter medicine, and opt for weight loss and exercise over expensive drugs or surgery. The choices you make, when combined with those of millions of others, will affect your health care costs.

PIPES EXPLODE

Back to our house: Emergencies happen.

The following winter you go on vacation. While you are gone, your pipes freeze and then burst. For two days, water runs freely throughout your house. The neighbor who watches your place calls you with the bad news. This time your insurance agent tells you your insurance will pay for all the repairs. Within minutes, you have a claims adjuster on the phone. The adjuster reminds you of your $500 deductible, but assures you that everything else is covered by insurance. Moments later, you notify your plumber. The adjuster recommends a general contractor that specializes in repairing water-damaged homes.

Even before you can catch a flight home, the plumber has turned off the water and the repair work has begun. Since you cannot stay in your house, the adjuster writes

29

you a check to cover your expenses at a very nice hotel near home.

Three weeks later you move back home, happy to sign over the $55,000 insurance check to the general contractor. You notice on the invoice that the plumber charged $18,000 for this work. This time you say, "Oh well, insurance is paying for it." Life is good again.

HUMAN PIPES RUPTURE

If your body's "pipes" rupture – you suffer a burst aorta, for instance – you do not worry about costs, the right surgeon, best hospital or extended care facility. You want your life saved. You dial 9-1-1 and could care less which ambulance company rushes you to the hospital. Weeks later, you are relieved that insurance covered it all, except for your $500 deductible. This is just like the way homeowner's insurance pays to repair your house. In either case, you really had no choice over whether to have the pipes repaired, and because insurance paid, you did not have to worry about cost.

Unfortunately, after your surgery, if you feel something leaking inside your body, it means more medical care and additional bills. Your insurance, however, will cover those costs, too.

When your body's "pipes" go bad, health care is not an optional purchase; you are grateful that your health care costs are paid by someone else, and you want no limits set on what it costs for you to regain your health.

If you never owned homeowners insurance and water destroyed your house, you could still move to an apartment and start over. If, on the other hand, your aorta bursts and your body is destroyed because of lack of health care, you are dead – there is no starting over.

Our health care system has given you many choices.

When the doctor spots something troubling, you choose between an X-ray that costs less or an MRI that costs more, depending on who pays for it. If insurance pays, you choose the MRI because you recognize its relative value – a better test at less cost to you. If insurance paid for your food, you would likely choose steak instead of hamburger – it is human nature.

In nations where government gatekeepers make health care decisions for you, you might want an MRI, but the gatekeeper sends you for an X-ray. You may have a bulging aorta, but a shortage of cardiovascular surgeons means waiting three months for surgery. When the gatekeeper controls your health care, you hope that when you get sick it will be a disease that places you at the head of the line, instead of in the waiting line.

The key feature of the U.S. health care system that impacts price more than any other is the fact that you do not personally pay much of the cost; through health insurance or a government program, someone else pays most of your health care bills.

WHY DOESN'T THE GOVERNMENT JUST DO SOMETHING TO REDUCE COST?

If cost is the overriding issue, you might ask, "Why doesn't the government just limit health care costs?"

Actually, they have tried to do this, through the Medicare and Medicaid systems. (Medicare is the federal government program that provides health care to people aged 65 and older. Medicaid's primary mission is to provide health care for low-income people younger than 65.) For an explanation of Medicare and Medicaid, and the new Medicare drug plan, read chapters eight and nine.

<u>Untold Truth</u>: The costs of government-provided health care are shifted to people who do not have government-provided health care.

The government has tried to hold down health care spending by price setting, which results in cost shifting. The government sets prices by limiting the amount it reimburses doctors, hospitals, and other providers for health care services.

Medicare and Medicaid reimbursements, the lowest payments that providers receive, are a fraction of what the provider really needs to charge to meet all the costs of those services. How do providers recover this lost revenue? They must receive larger reimbursements from workers who are not on a government program. Most of these workers are aged younger than 65, and receive health insurance through their employers.

Here is an example of cost-shifting. The doctor needs $200,000 to operate his clinic. Half of his patients are covered under Medicare, and the other half are not. His patients receive the same services. The government, however, will only reimburse the doctor $75,000 for his Medicare patients, so the doctor charges the non-Medicare patients $125,000. This is called cost-shifting. Just because Medicare limited the doctor's reimbursement rates does not mean they also reduced his costs, so he shifts those costs to non-Medicare patients.

Government funding of Medicare and Medicaid is something like playing with a balloon. If you squeeze one end of a balloon, the other end grows larger. Or if you squeeze the middle, both ends grow larger. Trying to force price controls onto health care is like squeezing that balloon from every direction. If squeezed too hard, it will eventually explode.

<u>Untold Truth</u>: Cost-shifting is one of the main reasons

why employers' health insurance premiums have suffered double-digit inflation during the past several years.

LOW PROVIDER REIMBURSEMENTS HAVE
NOT CONTROLLED HEALTH CARE SPENDING

Untold Truth: Overall spending has increased, because government-provided health care has created the perception that health care is free.

All types of government-provided health care accounted for 46 percent[6] of health care expenditures in 2003, though the government only insured 26 percent of the population.[7] This high spending was driven by high use. Those with government-paid health insurance – primarily Medicare and Medicaid – used more services.

Medicare enrollees, who also have a Medicare supplemental policy, pay nothing, or nearly nothing, for covered services. Medicaid patients pay very small co-payments (if any) for care. These users perceive that covered services are free. Since these services appear to be free, they are used more often. This is what drives up overall health care spending.

This higher spending forces increased costs onto employers and employees, because they pay the bulk of the costs through the Medicare payroll tax and other types of taxes. Many state budgets are in trouble because of runaway Medicaid costs, which have threatened other essential programs, like public education.

To pay for government health care programs, the government spent about $766 billion during 2003.[8]

Today's workers expect that when they turn age 65

6. "Table 1: National Health Expenditures Aggregate and Per Capita Amounts, and Average Annual Percent Growth, by Source of Funds, Selected Calendar Years: 1980-2003," CMS, Health and Human Services, U.S. Government.
7. "Table HI-1. Health Insurance Coverage Status and Type of Coverage by Sex, Race and Hispanic Origin: 1987 to 2004," CMS, Health and Human Services, U.S. Government 2.
8. See note 6.

they will have the same Medicare entitlements, or even more, than are available today. All their working lives they pay the Medicare tax, and they pay higher costs for medical services. They hope that tomorrow's younger workers will remain willing to pay their bills.

In the U.S., the government only spends 46 percent of the health care dollar. To know whether it would be wise to let the government control 100 percent of health care spending, we can look to foreign health care systems (see chapter 14).

MUCH MORE IS AT STAKE

"Still, we just cannot keep on spending so much on health care. We have to cut spending," you insist. More than one-seventh of our $11.1 trillion economy is spent on health care. Suppose we cut some of that and spent it on something else?

Before we tell the government to do something to cut health care spending, we need to understand what benefits it brings to us. We need to understand that more than our health is at stake.

U.S. health care is like a tapestry. You can readily see the colors and feel the texture of a tapestry on its surface. You can judge its beauty by simply looking at it, or touching it. What you cannot see without imagination is all that goes into making that tapestry: dyeing of the fabric and thread, weaving of the fabric, and sewing of each stitch. Seldom do people see the back side of a tapestry which can look chaotic, and even unattractive. Yet all of this is required to make a beautiful tapestry.

The jobs of millions of Americans are woven into the fabric of the United States health care tapestry. The cost of health care, like the selling price of a tapestry, is based on what can be seen, and what is hidden from view.

Stand in a hospital corridor and you see doctors, nurses, nurses' assistants, receptionists, ambulance drivers, shiny hospital floors, and stainless steel equipment. Not so easy to spot are the janitors who clean the buildings, clerks who process orders and file paperwork, hospital administrators, chaplains, and food handlers. Deep in the hospital's sub-basement works the engineer who operates the heating and air conditioning systems. You will never see the engineer, but his work is crucial to delivering your critical care upstairs in the emergency room.

Deeper into the health care tapestry, and unseen by patients, you find medical researchers who design equipment and drugs, manufacturers and their maintenance staff, security workers who protect their buildings, and the people who sell the drugs and equipment.

On the back side of the tapestry you find the attorneys who negotiate contracts and bring lawsuits, insurance sales and processing staff, banks, tradesmen who build the clinics and hospitals, food venders, auto workers who build ambulances, pavers who install and maintain parking lots, and the morticians who come at the very end of the health care system.

Mixed into the strange weave of the backside of the health care tapestry you find tens of thousands of government regulators, and those who pay the medical bills of the government's clients. Even the members of state legislatures and the U.S. Congress have stitched their way into the health care tapestry.

While you sit in the dentist's chair, you see only the top of the tapestry. You really have no idea how many jobs, directly and indirectly, are related to fixing your abscessed tooth. But all these workers are there, relying on you to pay for your root canal.

But there are even more jobs at stake.

The shiny pacemaker regulating the heartbeat of hundreds of thousands of people has a titanium case that begins when a miner digs a lump of iron ore out of the ground. Workers in Argentina drill the oil, brought to the United States on tankers staffed by seamen, that is processed by other workers into plastic for tubes, pill bottles, gloves and countless other medical products. An African diamond miner uncovers a shiny gem that becomes the tip of a drill used to expose the root in your tooth.

Our economy, and in many ways, the economies of many foreign nations, depends on a robust U.S. health care system. So do tens of millions of U.S. jobs. Artificially forcing down prices by government intervention will destroy jobs and damage economies; in the end, it would mean fewer health care services and higher unemployment.

The U.S. unemployment rates are consistently lower than those of foreign countries because we are a nation of workers and consumers. If foreign governments reduced some of their control over their economies and allowed people to spend more on health care voluntarily, they would have fewer unemployed workers.

WOW! HEALTH CARE PROVIDES ALL OF THIS?

"What do you mean that my indoor swimming pool isn't paid by my health insurance?" the indignant man asked. "I spent $25,000 on it, only because my doctor said I needed to swim every day due to the stiffness in the big toe on my right foot." This sounds ridiculous, but every experienced health insurance agent has heard such a statement at least once. People expect a lot from the health care system, and sometimes, they can be confused about what is covered.

The term "health care system" covers a huge range of services, products, and devices. Its primary purpose is to prevent and treat pain and suffering and extend people's lives. It works to improve the general health of all Americans, and it provides dignity of life to those who are chronically ill or dying. The health care system does this through a complex matrix of medical providers, and the costs are paid by a combination of insurance companies, governments, and private parties. The health care system expends more than $1.7 trillion[9] a year to pay all these costs.

How big is $1.7 trillion? If you took $100 bills and began to stack them tightly, $1 million would be about three feet tall. $1 billion would be about 3,000 feet tall. A stack of $100 bills that equaled $1 trillion would stand 630 miles high.[10] So, if all the money we in the U.S. spent on health care in 2003 – $1.7 trillion – could be stacked in a pile of $100 bills, it would reach 1,070 miles high – four times higher than the International Space Station; the distance between Kansas City and Philadelphia. That is a mountain of money! To spend it all, assuming that its value remained constant over time, you would need to purchase a $100 item every second of every day for 578 years.[11] Even Bill Gates could not do it.

Even before we are born, the health care system cares for our parents, making sure they are healthy and ready to birth a child. During pregnancy, Mom receives prenatal care and at delivery, the health care system provides a host of services to her and the baby.

Sick babies especially require very expensive and specialized care. In the United States, we do whatever we can to provide it. We do not spare any expense to give a tiny, sick baby a chance for life. This is not true in many foreign

9. Ibid.
10. Bob Vickers, *The Artful Askers Workbook*, National Heritage Foundation, February, 2005, 11.
11. Ibid.

nations where a government gatekeeper worries more about how much money is left in the budget. If funds are running short, so must the life of a baby at risk.

During our childhood and teen years, we receive a good deal of preventive care that continues on into adulthood. Our working years require care for illness. In fact, 80 percent of time lost on the job stems from illness, not accident. Job-related accidents, though, also consume a great deal of health care spending.

Transplants of human and artificial organs, heart surgery, dental and optical care, help us deal with our body's deterioration.

As we age, stiff muscles and joints become our daily companions, and sometimes they are debilitating. We need new knees or hips, a device to keep our heart beating, or a scooter to help us stay mobile.

For many Americans, chronic pain is a constant nag. To make life bearable, we take drugs, use medical devices, or receive special nursing care.

Then come our last few months. We ask the health care system to make them as comfortable as possible, and therein, health care spending spikes. As much as 80 percent or more of our lifetime health care costs occur during the last six months of life.

If our neighbor suffers from a deformity or disability, our caring nature requires the health care system to ease their way. If our children are born with severe disabilities, we want our institutions to do everything they can to give our child a chance at a good quality of life.

We have never tolerated a health care system like that of the Rumanians with their infamous orphanages, where abandoned children lived in tiny cribs in filthy rooms, with barely enough to survive. We never tolerated hospitals like those in Ukraine that cared for children who were victims of Chernobyl, leaving them to die from cancers in squalid facilities devoid of life-saving drugs, forcing their parents and family to provide for their basic needs. We would never let politics, graft and greed destroy the only medical clinic in our city as happened in Awka, Anambra State, Nigeria, a city of 152,000 people.

We ask a lot of our health care system. We demand that it be world class – even better than world class. We ask it to walk with us every moment of every day, whenever we get sick or injured. We want it to ease our pain and extend our life. We pay whatever it asks.

IF WE ARTIFICIALLY
DECREASE HEALTH CARE SPENDING

Let us suppose that we tell our elected officials through our votes and the messages they get from health care reformers, that we want them to find a way to cut our health care costs drastically.

Remember that currently, U.S. residents spend $1.7 trillion on health care in a year, or about 15.3 percent of our Gross Domestic Product. Many health care reformers think

Country	Percent of GDP	Savings if the U.S. Matched% of GDP
United States	15.3	– –
Germany	11.1	$466 billion
France	10.1	$577 billion
Canada	9.6	$633 billion
Japan	7.9	$821 billion
United Kingdom	7.7	$836 billion

that's too much, and want to see it reduced, more in line with foreign health care expenditures.

The chart on the previous page shows how much we would have to reduce our health care expenditures to meet the levels of spending common to these five, modern, government-controlled health care systems.

Suppose our government, like Germany, spent only 11.1 percent of GDP on health care, we would save $466 billion. Or 10.1 percent, like France: saving $577 billion. We could match Canada, saving $633 billion. Adopting Japanese health care might save us $821 billion (but we would also have to forgo beef for fish, and butter for fish oil). If we just matched the United Kingdom, we could save $836 billion. Wow! That would really free up some cash!

The most frightening and threatening events in life will occur if our health care system does not have adequate resources to care for us. If we transfer the power to control health care from the people to a government gatekeeper, and the government promises to cut $466 billion or more from our total health care bill, they must set a budget cap. Someone will lose services, and it will be the most vulnerable people: the aged, disabled, and sick babies.

The gatekeeper will decide against spending $60,000 to provide a 75-year old Grandma with an artificial hip, when that money could be used to provide a complete set of vaccines for 150 infants. The gatekeeper chooses not to spend $10,000 a month to provide care for a disabled person – $1.2 million every 10 years. If he can withhold spending like this for 10 people, the $12 million he saves will, instead, provide a complete set of vaccines for 30,000 children. The gatekeeper spends health care money in the most cost-effective manner because his funds are limited.

The politicians would have set a global health care expenditure cap, and that gatekeeper cannot exceed it.

The United States is the world's wealthiest nation. We are used to good incomes, maximum consumer choices, and the world's best health care. We spend 15.3 percent of GDP because we can. It may be that we cannot spend more than that, and it may be that we need to tighten our belts and spend less. The plain fact is that we could never have arrived at this point unless we had the money to do so. This is the fruit of our hard work. It's because of billions of dollars invested in our system by private parties, and our ability to spend discretionary dollars as we choose. All of this has fueled an explosion in medical technology and health care services.

Before we rush to Washington, D.C. and ask Congress to slash health care spending, let us answer these questions: Which of the health care services we now enjoy, and for what age groups or types of illnesses, are we willing to do without? And how much unemployment are we willing to tolerate? What will foreign citizens and we do without the medical innovations that stem from the United State's generous funding of medical research? What will third world nations do without the used, but still usable, equipment discarded by our system because of new technology?

THE MOST DIRECT WAY OF CONTROLLING HEALTH CARE SPENDING

We ask a lot of our health care system, and by how we live we often make its job even more difficult.

We drink too much alcohol and suffer liver damage. We eat too much and suffer high blood pressure. We love sweets and get diabetes. We smoke and get lung cancer.

We sleep too little and become mentally imbalanced.

41

We sleep and eat too much and become obese.

We go on a fad diet and lose 40 pounds, and then put 50 pounds back on.

We run long distances to lose weight and then suffer a heart attack. We become couch potatoes and suffer a heart attack. We eat the wrong kind of fats and get clogged veins and suffer a heart attack. We recover from a heart attack and then get lung cancer from smoking.

Americans may be willing to change their lifestyle to improve their health, but are we ready for a new national law telling us that we *must* do it!

CHAPTER 4
THE EVOLUTION OF THE MEDICAL REVOLUTION

It was 1903. Katherine felt the hard contractions that signaled the impending birth of her tenth child. She would deliver again in the isolated, rough wooden farmhouse that sat on the Oklahoma plains where she had birthed all of her children. The doctor arrived on horseback, and the family paid him with produce from their garden.

"Katherine's...doctor, who was in a hurry to get somewhere, gave her an overdose of ergot, a fungus used in those days to stimulate contractions. Katherine groaned in agony during her labor, yelling and crying from the severe pain of the forceful and hurried contractions. To keep her as comfortable as possible, they moved her from bed to chair and back to bed again. As the contractions continued to worsen, they created incredible pressure on her uterus, but Katherine's cervix had not yet dilated enough to release the baby. Finally, her uterus and abdomen ruptured in excruciating pain and she, along with the baby, died."[1]

Those were the "good old days" of health care.

---

1. Dave Racer, *To Change the Heart of Man*, To be released during 2006.

At the turn of the twentieth century, mothers served as the family's primary doctor; her home was the family hospital. Full-time professional doctors were scarce, and very overworked. Doctors knew their patients well, were inexpensive, had scant formal training, and very little medical information to help them improve their practice. In rural areas and smaller towns, they may also have been the town dentist or barber. Medical schools could only dream about training an army of specialists; there was neither the demand nor the money to do so. The primary care doctor did everything, which was very limited.

All this began to change rapidly in those years after Katherine lost her baby, as medical research and innovation exploded, aided by curious medical scientists and entrepreneurs, and a deluge of health care dollars.

THEN CAME THE MONEY

Before 1900, there were only about 200 hospitals in the United States, and most served low-income and indigent people. Then governments began licensing doctors and regulating hospitals. At the same time, the U.S. enjoyed unprecedented economic growth. Hospital construction exploded.

By the 1930s, despite the onrushing Great Depression, more than 7,000 hospitals were in business. In 1946, the federal government flooded the hospital system with hundreds of millions of dollars more, with the passage of the Hill-Burton Act. This law allowed hospitals to expand and modernize.

Today, after much consolidation, the total number of registered hospitals is about 5,759.[2]

---

2. "Fast Facts on U.S. Hospitals from AHA Hospital Statistics," hospitalconnect.com, 2006: http://www.aha.org/aha/resource_center/fastfacts/fast_facts_US_hospitals.html

To be successful, hospitals needed patients to fill their beds. Procedures previously done at home, or not done at all, now moved to the safer, sterile hospital.

During this same time, medical schools began in earnest to train doctors into specialties, and later, sub-specialties. They recruited the brightest and best students, and funded research that would lead to incredible health care breakthroughs.

These combined events drove four important health care changes: The quality of medical care increased rapidly. Life expectancy increased dramatically while infant mortality dropped. Governments invested heavily to improve public health (clean water, sewers, immunizations, divided highways, and such). The fourth change, the one that most of us are concerned about today, is that spending for health care services increased steadily.

Overseas, Germans saw their federal health care system, which began in 1883, expand to include more classes of people.

Russian Communists won a revolutionary war and began imposing a command economy on the people. Lenin called on Joseph Stalin to spread Communist philosophy to other nations. From the onset of Russian Communism, her leaders promised free, universal health care.

Japan implemented its national health care system in 1928. Other major nations that moved to government systems waited until after World War II to do so.

In 1912, President Theodore Roosevelt proposed a national health care system for the U.S., but Congress rejected it. Instead, we continued with a free market approach that birthed private health insurance. During the 1920s, Blue Cross offered coverage for catastrophic hospital expenses. This allowed people to pool their money so that if one of them got seriously ill or injured, insurance could help them pay their hospital bills. People who owned Blue Cross insurance paid 100 percent of their doctor and medicine bills. If they remained healthy, they would never have to file a claim or collect on their Blue Cross policies.

During a presidency that spanned from 1933 to 1945, Franklin Delano Roosevelt twice attempted to create a national health care system. U.S. citizens continued to reject it. President Harry Truman also promised to create a national health care system, but he, too, failed. The U.S. preferred a free market health care system.

In the late 1940s, Blue Shield began offering high deductible catastrophic insurance to pay doctor bills. Most Blue Shield and Blue Cross premiums were paid by employers as a benefit to employees. Other insurance companies began to compete with the "Blues." The free market continued to respond to the wishes of U.S. voters as they rejected a federal government takeover of health care.

During the 1940s and 50s, when a patient used health care services, they paid the doctor and collected the receipts. They knew what the doctor charged. When the receipts were added together, they seldom exceeded the policy deductible. The greatest majority of Americans, even those with Blue Shield insurance, paid for all their doctor care and "medicine" out of their own pocket. Insurance costs were low, because claims were few.

In chapter seven we look at health insurance – how it works, who pays, and why it has become so expensive. The fact is, the trillions of dollars paid by insurance companies and government agencies during the past 80 years to medical providers has fueled a revolution in health care quality that rivals all of human history.

ASTOUNDING MEDICAL BREAKTHROUGHS

In 1951, Americans read about Dr. John Lewis performing successful open-heart surgery – the first successful operation of its kind in the world. This opened the floodgates to more and increasingly complex heart procedures. Cardiovascular surgery became a medical specialty. The heart-lung machine and trained cardiovascular surgeons eventually made open-heart surgery common.

In 1957, Earl Bakken delivered his new heartbeat-regulating device to Dr. C. Walton Lillihei, and the doctor implanted it in a baby. The pacemaker had begun to extend lives, and eventually gave birth to the Medtronic Corporation, a leader of the medical device industry.

Doctors began preferring the more lucrative and prestigious specialty practices and by the late 1950s, some feared a great shortage of general practitioners. Those most concerned about this created a new specialty, the family practice doctor, to be the generalist that met the patient before they went to specialists.

In 1965, Congress created Medicare and Medicaid. This infused billions of dollars annually into the provision of health care services for older U.S. residents, and for low-income citizens.

The world learned that on December 3, 1967, Dr. Christiaan Barnard had transplanted a new heart into 53-year-old Lewis Washkansky. Though Washkansky lived only 18 more days, this feat fueled a wave of innovative human organ transplant surgeries. Others worked toward the creation of artificial organs to replace the sparse number of human organs available for transplant.

In 1972, Wall Street applauded the explosion in price of the stock of a medical device company. Minneapolis-based Bio-Medicus, Inc., which had opened at $5.00 a share in January, shot to more than $87 a share by September, because of the news of a breakthrough in artificial heart technology. This had happened despite the fact that

Bio-Medicus had never sold a single product.[3] Investors recognized that they stood to make millions if the company could perfect and sell a workable artificial heart. Capitalists had seized on the astounding profits to be made from health care innovation.

In 1982, Dr. John Najarian performed a successful liver transplant on 11-month-old Jamie Fisk. Najarian went on to develop a highly effective drug that fought off the deadly effects of the body's immune system. Also in 1982, surgeons implanted the Jarvik-7 artificial heart into Barney Clark.

Transplants provide a great example of how medical costs multiply. So that Najarian could even attempt the liver transplant, millions of dollars were first spent on research and animal experimentation. To get a human body to accept a transplanted organ, "super drugs" such as Najarian's ALG had to be invented. The research and development of those 1970s specialized drugs cost tens of millions of dollars. Those costs were paid by patients and eventually, by insurance.

Penicillin first became available for use by doctors during the early 1940s.[4] Within a few decades, drug companies seemed to roll out new, powerful miracle drugs each month. By 2004, the cost of developing a new wonder drug soared to more than $900 million (see chapter 10).

We became enthralled by seemingly daily news reports of new drugs, medical devices, and surgical breakthroughs – labeled experimental medicine. During the 1970s, very little of the cost of experimental medicine was paid by insurance.

As news media began to publicize the plight of individuals who had been denied a life-saving treatment, politi-

---

3. See note 1.

4. Mary Bellis, "The History of Penicillin,"
http://inventors.about.com/library/inventors/blpenicillin.htm

cians and the insurance companies felt the pressure to cover an increasing number of new procedures. Soon insurance began to pay for open-heart surgery, transplants, medical devices, and drug routines that had previously not been covered – experimental medicine became a mandated insurance benefit. State legislatures passed other laws that mandated scores of benefits to be covered by insurance. All of this had the effect of driving up the cost of health insurance premiums.

ENTITLEMENT BECAME COMMON

From the 1940s, when hardly anyone had health insurance, to 60 years later, our perception of who should pay medical bills has changed radically. According to the federal government, by 2003, all but 14 percent of the total cost of health care was paid either by government-provided insurance or private health insurance.

In 1973, Congress created a new type of health care delivery system – the Health Maintenance Organization (HMO). HMOs emphasized preventive care, and provided sick care. You could have regular physicals, and take your children to the doctor for common colds and other minor illnesses. Instead of paying for care each time you saw the doctor, your premiums pre-paid the health care provider. Doctors were paid whether or not you used their services. With HMOs, the United States had moved from low-premium, catastrophic health insurance, to high-premium, pre-paid health plans – and we were not shy about using those services.

By emphasizing preventive care, the HMO believed you would stay healthier for a longer time. By staying healthier, they believed that your lifetime health care costs would be reduced. These new, comprehensive services attracted large numbers of young families as premium-payers. Younger people had not yet developed a long-term relationship with a family doctor, and did not mind a clinic setting in which they might see a different doctor each time they visited.

HMOs also knew that preventive services are the least expensive form of health care. It had, however, some unintended results. Medical conditions that had previously gone undetected were found during routine physicals. This resulted in the need for additional health care services. Those younger families began to age, resulting in more health problems that needed attention. The consumption – called utilization – of health care increased. Patients perceived that their pre-paid health care plans entitled them to additional services at no additional cost.

Meanwhile, older and less healthy persons wanted preventive care, lab tests and the like, but they wanted to maintain their relationship with their family doctor. They opted for traditional health insurance plans, but demanded more benefits, like those offered by HMOs. Forced to offer nearly unlimited services to their less healthy policyholders, the insurance companies regularly increased their premiums. Many traditional insurance companies pulled out of the health insurance market altogether, unable to offer the comprehensive services and lower premiums offered by HMOs. Meanwhile, some insurance agents moved their less healthy groups to HMOs to take advantage of lower rates and more services.

By the mid-1980s, HMO and traditional insurance premiums had begun to feel expensive. By then, however, most U.S. residents owned some form of health insurance or belonged to an HMO. Premium cost, however, had left some people unable to afford HMO-type policies. Thus, politicians took up the cause of the uninsured, fueling a heated national debate.

Until the 1940s, nearly _every_ United States resident had been _uninsured_, but by the 1980s, the idea had taken hold that being uninsured was the same as living without health care.

From 1960, when individuals paid 47 percent of health care costs out of their own pocket,[5] by 2003, various forms of insurance had reduced out-of-pocket costs to just 13 percent.[6] Those costs, however, had sky-rocketed.

COSTS EXPLODED

By 1980, the total spent on U.S. health care had ballooned to $245.8 billion and consumed about 8.8 percent of GDP.[7] Those billions of dollars that U.S. residents spent on health care in the 1980s worried the insurance companies, HMOs, and government agencies that paid the bills. The media announced that once again a "health care crisis" had unfolded. Insurance premiums had spiraled upward, and researchers announced that millions of people were uninsured (see chapter 13).

Government policymakers began wringing their hands. The talk about creating a national health care system resurfaced. When Ronald Reagan became president, the march toward a national health care system, run by government-gatekeepers, quieted down.

During the late 1980s and early 1990s, the media reported a continuous increase in the number of uninsured U.S. residents. As a result, individual states began under-

---

5. "National Health Expenditures by Type of Service & Source of Funds: Calendar Years 2004-1960," Centers for Medicare & Medicaid Services, U.S. Government, 3.

6. Ibid., 1.

7. "Table 1, National Health Expenditures Aggregate and per Capita Amounts, Percent Distribution, and Average Annual Percent Growth, by Source of Funds: Selected Calendar Years, 1980-2003," United States, Centers for Medicare and Medicaid Services.

writing health care costs for many of their residents, so that even some middle class families qualified for taxpayer-subsidized insurance.

In 1992, U.S. voters elected Bill Clinton as their forty-second president and soon after, the health care crisis once again became front-page news. The U.S. Census Bureau announced that more than 15 percent of U.S. residents were now uninsured. Washington, D.C. policymakers began a very well-publicized search for the solution to this crisis.

In 1993, U.S. residents spent $888 billion on health care, 13.3 percent of GDP.[8] First Lady Hillary Clinton took the lead for national health care reform, calling together a group of experts from across the country. For months, they met in secret to devise the solution to our health care crisis.

When Mrs. Clinton's group finally released their suggestions, it came in the form of a 1368-page bill in Congress.[9] United States voters soundly rejected this new effort. Her plan had proposed a federal government-gatekeeper health care system much like that of Germany (see chapter 19). Mrs. Clinton's health care plan may have directly led to the Republicans gaining control of Congress after the 1994 election. By their votes, Americans had again let it be known that they did not want the federal government to take over health care; they preferred the free market approach.

Despite this forceful rejection of a national health care system, our problems with the cost of health care have continued to trouble us. Once again, early in the twenty-first century, we have another "health care crisis." By 2003, the total dollar amount spent on U.S. health care had ballooned to $1.7 trillion, and consumed 15.3 percent of GDP:[10] 45

---

8. Ibid.

9. H.R. 3600, 103rd Congress, 1994.

10. See note 7.

million of us are, allegedly, uninsured.

SPENDING BECAUSE WE WANT IT

U.S. residents as a whole spend a lot of money on health care because we are a wealthy nation.

Millions of middle-class Americans think nothing of spending $25,000 on a new car, or $350,000 for a home, or $50,000 for a college education. Likewise, we spend hundreds or even thousands of dollars a month as we insure our lives, health, autos, homes, collectors' items, businesses, and even more.

When we rear-end another car and damage our front end, we take our car to the best repair shop in town. We want the body man and mechanic to fix everything so that it will look and run even better than before the accident. We expect our insurance to pay the $3,000 bill, even though we first have to shell out $500 for the deductible. "At least I'm getting something back for that $1250 insurance premium I pay every year," we tell the repairman, who does not let us drive away until he has been paid in full.

We expect our health insurance to work in much the same way.

We want access to the best doctors whom we can trust; we want hospitals where high quality treatment is available; we want medical devices to help us overcome disabilities created by birth, disease, or accident; we want to receive therapy so that we can return to work; we want drugs to help us live longer and more comfortably, while avoiding critical diseases and managing pain.

None of us want to buy our medical services from "Discount Doctors, Inc." or get our surgeries done at "Susie's Surgical Warehouse." When we are sick, we want quick access to a doctor who will do whatever we need to get well.

We expect others to share our health care costs with us. If we work for a company, we want our employers to pay for most of our health insurance. We want our co-pays and deductibles to be low. And we want the freedom to go to the doctor, hospital, or clinic of our choice.

BUT IT HAS PAID OFF

All that we spend on health care, and health care insurance, has paid off in many ways.

> "The caveman was lucky to hit his 20s. A compound fracture, appendicitis, or even an abscessed tooth could mean a sure and painful death. In the times of Charlemagne the life expectancy was about 35 years. *In the United States, in 1910 one could expect to live to 50 years.* Now, at the turn of the millennium, our life expectancy is [78] years, with women outliving men by about 6-7 years."[11] [Emphasis added]

Residents of the United States have seen their life expectancy constantly increase during the last 100 years.

> "The increase is mostly due to medical advances (such as immunizations and antibiotics), public health measures, indoor plumbing, and healthier lifestyles...With optimum lifestyles, we can now reasonably expect an active life until 85 or late 80s. People over 85

---

11. Glenn R. Stout, M.D., "How to Stack the Deck in Your Favor," 2000, Senior FAA Medical Examiner, http://www.cami.jccbi.gov/AAM-400A/FASMB/HOP/longevity.htm.

now make up the fastest-growing segment of our population. A baby born today has about one chance in 25 to become a centenarian."[12]

People who, in years past, had been bedridden now drive cars, have motorized wheel chairs and active lives. When age has dimmed our eyesight, surgery restores to us a quality of vision like that of a teenager. Those with bad kidneys, livers, hearts, or other diseased organs, receive transplants or medical devices that give them many more years of life. Crippling pain, diabetes, high blood pressure, and more, are controlled by miracle drugs. Devices regulate pain, heartbeat, and insulin.

The extraordinarily good U.S. health care system we enjoy today was created by human ingenuity fueled by trillions of dollars. The 15.3 percent of GDP that we spend on health care is the fuel that drives new discoveries that reduce suffering while extending life.

From doctors on horseback, we have gotten to Medevac helicopters that deliver patients to acute care hospitals within minutes of a serious accident. Even while on the way, Emergency Medical Technicians deliver life-saving care.

Patients with an abscessed tooth no longer go to the town barber to get it pulled; they sit in a comfortable chair, take a sedative, and 30 minutes later have gained relief from physical pain (but face financial pain to pay for their root canal), and the dentist saves their tooth.

Medical specialists, who were almost non-existent in 1900 now practice medicine in their own fully equipped, modern clinics and surgical centers. They compete with the hospitals for patients.

---

12. Ibid.

Never before in the history of mankind has there been such an abundance of high-quality health care for so many people as there is in the U.S.

Americans have decided, through their pocketbooks and their votes, that they will not settle for third-world health care: what they want is to ensure that they can continue to expect first-class health care services and be able to afford them.

Doctors sit in the middle of the health care system, refereeing between the insurance companies that pay the costs, patients who expect high quality, and the trial lawyers who wait for them to make a mistake. Doctoring, like the health care system, has come a long way since Dr. Welby.

CHAPTER 5
CALLING
DR. WELBY

Myth: Doctors' high salaries are the reason that U.S. health care costs so much.

To some, Marcus Welby, MD, the family doctor in the popular TV series that aired from 1969-1976, represents the "golden age" of doctoring.

After high school, Welby spent four years in college, three years in medical school and a year as an intern. As an intern, Welby worked 110-hour weeks.

He became a general practitioner – GP. Some of his medical school friends wanted to specialize instead of being GPs, so they entered residencies – gaining advanced training in surgery, OB-GYN, urology, or even sub-specialties like neuro-, cardiovascular, or plastic surgery.

Dr. Welby worked 75 to 90-hour weeks, and earned more money than most of his patients, but he had less time to spend it. He remained on call nearly all the time, and a good part of his day found him making house calls. When he saw a patient, it usually was because they were ill and could not come to his office. Even those who came to his office usually did so because they were sick. Almost no one came for preventive care.

Welby's community held him in high esteem. Patients took his advice, usually without question. A Welby patient would *never* sue a doctor.

Welby worked in a clinic that he owned. He set his own prices and made all the decisions about patient care.

Patients paid him either at the time of an office call, or soon after. He provided quite a bit of charity care, and if the local economy slowed, he forgave many debts.

He referred his patients to the local hospital, where he "had privileges," meaning that he also performed some of his medical procedures in a hospital setting. The hospital offered the general population a good range of services. Welby could send the tough cases to the university medical school.

Marcus Welby, MD sacrificed normal family life. He made hospital rounds before morning's first light, and saw patients all day. He knew each of his patients and their families, served them for decades, and had ample time to talk to them about health issues.

Dr. Welby strongly encouraged his own children to go into medicine. By the time he semi-retired in 1985, however, the health care system had experienced radical changes that discouraged him about the future of doctoring.

Today, Marcus Welby is more likely to be Martha Wilson, a dermatologist, who is married to Mike Smith, a pathologist, and both of them work for a multi-practice clinic owned by a large corporate medical provider. Their work week of 40-50 hours allows them a relatively normal home life in the suburbs. Dr. Wilson's patients come to her, and during her career, she has handled only a small number of emergency calls.

How Dr. Wilson practices medicine is greatly determined by what is covered by Medicare, Medicaid, or health insurance; she is diligent to follow their best practice guidelines. Doctors and other health professionals have developed these guidelines, also called evidence-based or best-science medicine, to provide physicians with treatment protocols. They are meant to hold down the overall cost of providing health care by guiding the doctor toward the most successful tests and procedures, while avoiding those shown to be ineffective or unnecessary. The guidelines also provide health care managers with a way to evaluate the doctor's performance.

Though they have a great income and reasonable hours, their personal satisfaction from the job of doctoring has diminished, so Drs. Martha and Mike decided to encourage their children to become computer systems specialists, or go into business for themselves. These are the sobering questions they ask themselves, and their children ask them: "Why would any intelligent person choose a profession where income is guaranteed to fall 30 percent over the next five years, where your every action is second-guessed by government or health plans, where malpractice suits are a constant worry, and where you are blamed at every turn for the exorbitant cost of care? Why would any rational, business-minded physician accept Medicare or Medicaid payment below their costs of doing business? Why indeed?"[1]

GETTING THAT M.D. DEGREE

It takes many years of study and practice before a student can hang a Doctor of Medicine degree on his or her wall, and several more before they finally become board certified. Board certification means that the doctor has

1. Richard L. Reece, M.D., *Voices of Health Care Reform, Options for Repackaging American Health Care*, Practice Support Resources, Inc., 2005, 207.

completed a vigorous and difficult course of study, completed months and years of practice, and has passed oral and written exams.

Their education begins with four years of college, with heavy emphasis on "...undergraduate work in physics, biology, and inorganic and organic chemistry."[2] Pre-med students also take "...courses in English, other humanities, mathematics, and the social sciences..."[3] to help them be well-rounded professionals.

Before completing a Bachelor of Science degree, the pre-med student begins applying to a medical school. "There are 144 medical schools in the United States."[4] About 35 percent of those who apply to a U.S. medical school will be admitted. Medical school will take four years, two of which will be academics, theory, and the law pertaining to medicine. During the second two years, they work with patients under the watchful eye of an experienced teaching doctor.

As they hang their M.D. certificate on the wall, they face the repayment of student loans of $100,000-$150,000. Yet, there is still more training ahead.

During medical school, the intern begins the application process for a specialty practice. Their specialty choice will determine their future lifestyle. For those, like Drs. Martha and Mike, who want relatively normal lives, specialties such as dermatology, pathology, or anesthesiology are great choices. They pay well and offer relatively normal working hours, with very little on-call work.

Today, the term "primary care physician" has different names. These may be general practitioner, family physi-

---

2. "Derm Career," American Board of Dermatology, 2005.

3. Ibid.

4. Ibid.

cian, OB-GYN, pediatrician, or general internist. The general practitioner may or may not be board certified.

On the other end of the scale are specialists who work in critical-care settings where urgent medical complications require highly developed skills and long workweeks – i.e., emergency medicine, trauma surgery, etc.

Some doctors still choose solo or small group practices in clinics they own. These require them to wear the many hats of a small business operator in addition to staying current in their specialty. In fact, "80% of doctors practice in groups of 10 or less."[5]

During their residencies, doctors are paid a modest salary: perhaps $25,000-$30,000 per year. They still have education and other living costs, so they usually accumulate more debt.

Those who enter a specialty face four to ten years or more of additional training, and may spend another one to two years in practice before they can take the tests required to become board certified. When you see a framed certificate on your doctor's wall that says he or she is certified by the American Board of Ophthalmology, for instance, you will know that it represents years of hard, disciplined study and practice.

Some doctors turn 40 before entering private practice, after a dozen years of residency. These highly trained doctors will never be like Drs. Martha and Mike; instead, they will work long hours, both in the office and on call.

The doctor's practice is watched closely by hospital administrators, government regulators, and insurance company managers, and they feel the pressure of the trial lawyers who always are one slip-of-the-finger away from threatening their status and livelihood. These specialists

---

5. See note 1, 208.

will, however, earn very high incomes during their short-ened working life.

U.S. culture rewards highly trained specialists in near-ly all occupations, whether that specialist is an orthopedic surgeon with 16 years of college, graduate and post-graduate schooling, or a Chicago teenager with extreme basketball skills. Since there are few of either of these, both are well paid, but one might agree that the athlete is paid out of proportion to their real value to society.

HIGH DEBT, SHORT CAREERS

The work life and financial rewards of a highly skilled surgeon are something like that of a professional athlete, only reversed.

Duke University heavily recruited Jack Jones[6] out of a Chicago high school. He made all-American as a sopho-more and left college after two years, signing a three-year, $5 million guaranteed contract with an NBA team. He worked hard, became all-pro, and in his fourth year, signed a five-year, $75 million contract. During this time, howev-er, the physical demands he made of his legs, knees, and hips slowed him down. Finally, suffering from hip and knee problems, Jones retired at age 32. He was faced with trying to live on less than $15 million a year.

To be able to pay Jones' $15 million salary meant that tens of thousands of fans had to purchase tickets to home games, watch away games on TV, and purchase the adver-tisers' and sponsors' products. This money comes from Americans' discretionary income, the same pool of money that has fueled our world-class health care system.

At age 38, our retired basketball player had difficulty walking. Jack Jones needed knee replacement surgery.

---

6. Fictitious name. Any relation to a real person is strictly coincidental.

Jones sought out 38-year old Dr. Pete Pollard, a board certified orthopedic surgeon to whom he was referred by the team trainer. Dr. Pollard worked in a specially designed and equipped orthopedic surgical center located near the affluent suburbs in which most of the professional athletes lived.

Dr. Pollard, who still owed $180,000 in student loans, hoped to pay off his college debt by age 45. After that, he hoped to experience not only the joy of helping old basketball players walk again, but the security offered by a high income – maybe even get time to play golf.

Dr. Pollard scored a "slam dunk" during surgery, restoring the knee so well that Jones considered making a comeback. The insurance company paid all the costs of Jones' new knee, a good chunk of which found its way into Dr. Pollard's paycheck.

The surgical center had heavily recruited Dr. Pollard while he was a resident. They offered him a generous salary and income incentives, so that soon his total compensation exceeded $300,000 a year.

When Jack Jones hit 55, he had his first hip replacement. Dr. Pollard also performed this surgery. By then, the doctor had accumulated a multi-million dollar investment portfolio, and though still relatively young, considered retirement. The stress from complying with government regulations and practice guidelines had sapped his idealism. Worse yet, a retired football player had sued him for $10 million in a malpractice suit, and he didn't want to go through that again.

During his medical practice, Dr. Pollard had very little time to spend with his wife and children. He, like 64 percent of doctors his age,[7] strongly urged his college-age children to do something other than doctoring.

---

7. Merritt, Hawkins & Associates, "2004 Survey of Physicians 50 to 65 Years Old, Based on 2003 Data," http://www.merritthawkins.com/pdf/2004_physician50_survey.pdf

WHAT DOCTORS EARN

When a doctor makes a mistake in judgment, people suffer physical pain, lifetime disability, or even die. This is why we require so much training of them. It is also why they are well paid.

What we pay a doctor depends on numerous factors. Geographical location, specialty, education, and experience – supply and demand – will set their compensation. A doctor's total compensation is a reflection of the income he or she can generate for a clinic, practice group, or hospital employer. That income comes from patient fees, consultation fees, lab tests, medical procedures, and even the sale of medical products and devices.

Doctors in lower-risk specialties who prefer 40-50 hour workweeks will earn less than the entrepreneurs and risk-takers who have highly developed skills, and years of training. The perceived risk and complexity of a doctor's specialty will affect their compensation.

The table on the next page reflects the average annual compensation earned by various physician specialists (in practice for at least three years).

Neurosurgeons make $424,000 a year. Does that seem about right, too much, or too little? Your answer may depend on whether you are about to have surgery. During brain surgery, you wouldn't want to hear the surgeon say, "Oops. Snipped the wrong synapse. Oh well."

That is why we pay neurosurgeons so much, and why we are glad that health insurance pays their bills.

WHY ARE DOCTORS GLUM?

Doctors are able to earn high incomes during their years of practice. They also must spend a great deal of

Specialty[8]	Avg. Compensation
Family Practice	150,000
Pediatrics[9]	149,754
OB-GYN	247,000
Otolaryngology	304,000
Cardiology	320,000
General Surgery	255,000
Gastroenterology	298,000
Hospitalist	171,000
Neurosurgery	424,000
Neurology	209,000
Orthopedic Surgery	361,000
Dermatology[10]	232,000
Psychiatry	176,000
Anesthesiology	303,000
Radiology	355,000
Emergency Medicine[11]	211,880
Internal Medicine	161,000
Urology	329,000
Pathology[11]	254,800

8. Merritt, Hawkins & Associates, "Summary Report, 2005 Review of Physician Recruitment Incentives," http://www.merritthawkins.com/pdf/2005_incentive_survey.pdf

9. "Physician Compensation Salary Survey, in Practice Three Plus Years," http://www.physicianssearch.com/physician/salary2.html, June 30, 2005.

10. Ibid.

11. An average computed from: http://www.merritthawkins.com/pdf/2004_modernhealthcare_comp_review.pdf

money to stay current, pay business and insurance expenses, and conform to countless regulations enforced on them by governments, hospitals, clinics, HMOs, and insurance companies. They also must worry about medical malpractice (see chapter 6).

The life of a physician brings some of the greatest satisfaction known to mankind, and some of the worst sorrow. Except for a pastor or priest, no other professional is so engrafted into the most powerful moments of real human drama. This is why people become doctors, why the practice of medicine appeals to idealists. High incomes are, of course, also a well-received and desirable benefit.

"Doctors in earlier generations rarely even spoke to each other about business. It wasn't necessary. They were going to make a decent living no matter what their business skills. They were paid fully for claims they submitted. They didn't ask permission to perform a procedure, refer a patient, or hospitalize a patient."[12]

Those earlier doctors chose treatments from among a few drugs, a small number of surgical options, two or three diagnostic tests, and very limited patient information. Today, their choices are complicated and at the same time, enhanced by a dozen or more drugs, many surgical options, and several diagnostic tests. The internet has armed patients with knowledge that results in questions, demands, and challenges to which the modern doctor must respond intelligently and often, forcefully.

As Medicare, Medicaid, HMOs and other forms of managed care came to dominate the delivery of health care, doctors had to grapple with something new: others telling them how to practice. They had no choice but to listen, since following practice guidelines determined whether, and how much, they would be paid. In essence, the method

---

12. Richard L. Reece, M.D., "For Young Doctors, It's Not Marcus Welby's Practice," 2005.

and amount of reimbursement began to direct medical care decisions.

Doctors resent third party insurance clerks, politicians, and trial lawyers determining how they practice medicine. They prefer to practice their art, not be forced to make medical decisions based on financial considerations. We patients, likewise, want doctors to do whatever it takes to solve our medical problems, reduce our pain, and extend our lives. Money, we feel, should be the least important part of the decision, especially when insurance pays the bills.

"Go into any medical staff room. You'll hear more talk about business concerns than clinical medicine. This should come as no surprise. Malpractice costs are soaring, practice costs are rising at four times the rate of income, and doctors are spending more time treating aging patients with more complex diseases at lower reimbursement rates."[13]

The low reimbursement rates paid by Medicare and Medicaid mean that each day doctors must see far more patients than they prefer. It is how they can keep enough cash flowing to pay all the bills. This means that they have to limit the amount of time they spend with each patient, and neither they nor their patients like this at all.

U.S. doctors aged 50 or older are often discouraged and frustrated. "Over three quarters (76%) of physicians [over 50] surveyed indicated that in the last five years they have found the practice of medicine to be less satisfying, while only 9% found it to be more satisfying."[14] Because of this, more than half of them hope to be able to change the way they practice medicine, cutting back on patients, and in some cases, retiring early.

---

13. Ibid.
14. See note 7.

SHORTAGES LOOM

The price and availability of health care is still subject to the law of supply and demand. During the next 20-40 years, this could become painfully evident. The current demand for health care services will be fueled by the medical problems faced by 79 million baby boomers as they enter their senior years. Baby boomers are the generation born between 1946 and 1964.

"The nation now has about 800,000 active physicians, up from 500,000 20 years ago."[15] Still, not enough men and women are entering the medical profession to keep up, and too many are retiring early.

"In February, 2002, the journal Health Affairs published a study by the Medical College of Wisconsin predicting a shortage of 200,000 physicians by the year 2020." Other, more conservative estimates, predict, "a shortage of 96,000 physicians by the year 2020."[16]

Doctors are paid well, compared to other professionals. So, income has little to do with those factors that turn young people away from medical careers. Job satisfaction, expensive and lengthy educational requirements, long hours, short working life, the cost of malpractice insurance, and the constant threat of lawsuits have compounded the problem. Whereas in the recent past some experts have complained that there are too many U.S. doctors, there is now general agreement that a shortage of doctors looms.

Unlike an auto factory that can plow ground today, build a modern assembly plant, and see cars rolling out in less than two years, "assembling" a doctor takes 15-20 years. To allay that predicted shortfall means that those

---

15. Dennis Cauchon, "Medical miscalculation creates doctor shortage. After a glut was predicted a decade ago, the number of physicians isn't keeping up with the demands of a wealthy, aging population," *USA TODAY*, Feb. 3, 2005.
16. See note 7.

future doctors should be in medical school today – and they are not.

The 1994 health care plan advanced by First Lady Hillary Clinton would have magnified the problem. Her plan stated that the number of doctors, "shall be reduced..."[17] The percentage of the mandatory reduction was to be decided by a national council, whose members were to be appointed by the secretary of health and human services (HHS). The president, of course, would appoint the secretary.

Reducing the number of doctors in training posed a problem for the medical schools and residency programs that trained them. Specifically, they stood to lose a lot of money. So the Clinton bill planned to pay the schools not to train doctors, just as the government pays farmers not to grow corn, allocating at least $23.2 billion during the first five years.[18] In addition, because fewer patients would be treated in these programs, academic health centers (hospitals and clinics) would also lose money. So, the government planned to pay them at least $17 billion not to treat patients.[19] Of the $40.2 billion needed to pay for these two programs, at least $8 billion would have been taken out of Medicare trust funds.[20] The balance would be paid by assessments charged to the new Regional Health Alliances, who would have gotten their money from your insurance premiums.

Mrs. Clinton believed that by artificially limiting the number of doctors, the government could control health

17. H.R. 3600, 103rd Congress, 1994, 513, lines 9-11.

18. Ibid., lines 8-15, 519.

19. Ibid., 553-554.

20. Ibid., 747-748. This number equals the minimum payments to be made under the law for the first five years of the program. The actual cost is determined by a formula that accounts for increases in the Consumer Price Index and other factors. The total amount transferred from Medicare funds would have been far greater than $8 billion over the course of time had Congress passed this bill.

spending, maybe even reduce it. Had Congress and U.S. voters accepted her plan, the shortages now projected for 2020 would be far worse. This, as much as anything, is a strong indicator why people suffer when the government is the health care gatekeeper.

The free market can find ways to adjust to some of the doctor shortage by finding efficiencies, reducing duplicative services, shedding unnecessary tests, creating new drug therapies, putting caps on malpractice lawsuits, and improving surgical technology. The shortage of U.S. doctors, however, is a critical problem made worse by government interference.

OTHER TYPES OF MEDICAL PROFESSIONALS IN MAINLINE MEDICINE

One of the ways the free market responds in the U.S. is to train non-physicians as medical professionals that provide a great deal of care at reduced cost.

Physician assistants, working under the supervision of a medical doctor, perform many of the same procedures as do the MDs. They typically have completed a four-year college degree, a certified physician assistant course similar to medical school, and must pass a national certification program. Some medical establishments consider PAs to be physician extenders. This allows an MD to accomplish more by assigning some of their workload to the PA. To the patient, the PA looks, acts, and practices just like an MD, except that he or she must always defer to the direction of the supervising physician.

Nurse practitioners and advance practice nurses likewise do many of the same tasks as medical doctors. Nurse midwives, who often work for their own clinics, deliver thousands of babies each year. Nurse anesthetists, working under the supervision of an anesthesiologist – a medical doctor – often care for patients during surgery.

These types of medical professionals serve to increase the quantity and quality of services. Highly trained physicians still lead the practice of medicine, but can extend their effectiveness while holding down overall costs by working with these other skilled medical professionals. For you, it means that your health care dollars can stretch farther without sacrificing quality.

Some of the factors that drive up the cost of health care are hidden from view. Among the most difficult of these is the pressure doctors feel from the invisible hand of a trial lawyer, waiting to sue them for malpractice.

CHAPTER 6
DOCTORS
PLAYING DEFENSE

One of the authors had an electrocardiogram during February of 1991, which he discussed with his doctor. The prior day, he had suffered a series of "flutters" in his chest.

"Well, I think you should have a stress test," his doctor said.

"Oh," he said. "How much does that cost?"

"Huh?" asked his doctor, who seldom heard such a question. "Oh, I suppose about $400 or $500."

"Well, I don't have health insurance," he said, being between jobs.

"Well, you really don't need the test," the doctor said, matter-of-factly. "I just thought it would help you feel better and worry less." He told him to relax, get more exercise and sleep, "and you need to lose weight." The doctor had told the truth, since this author is still alive and living flutter-free.

He had seen the same doctor for most of his adult life, and had a good doctor-patient relationship. Still his doctor worried about the potential of making a mistake. A mistake, the doctor knew, could cost the author his health, and put the doctor at risk of a medical malpractice lawsuit. The doctor really did not want to risk it. Doing the test could offer protection for both the doctor and patient.

Today's computer-savvy, internet-addicted patient might respond differently. "Doctor, I found a number of websites that say a fluttering sensation in the chest is an early indicator of heart disease, and it is highly suggested that you give me an electrocardiogram and send me for a nuclear stress test right away." If the doctor agrees to these tests, they will cost approximately $115 for the EKG, and $1,000 for the stress test.[1]

The other author, who did have insurance, had a 16-year-old son who kept waking up in the middle of the night with shortness of breath. After two nights without sleep as he worried about his son, the other author decided to make a direct trip to Children's Hospital. Due to the strong relationship he enjoyed with the son's pediatrician, he talked to the doctor by 8:45 a.m., and the doctor knew that no matter what he said, that son would be on his way to the hospital. "Well, I think you should go to Children's and have an echogram. I'll call and set it up," the doctor offered. (That echogram could cost $1,700 or more today.)[2]

The father suggested that he wanted the cardiologist who would read it to have grey hair, wanting an experienced doctor to care for his son. "Then I want an immediate consultation after the test is done," the father said. He did not want to have to go back to the pediatrician to get results.

By 11:30 a.m., the cardiologist had met with the father and explained that the son had a normal heart, and that his symptoms were common among young athletes.

---

1. Prices based on estimate provided by the Heart Institute of the Cascades, for 2005, via email to the author on 11/21/05, and will vary depending on location, exact procedure and other factors.
2. Ibid.

What doctor who wants to avoid a lawsuit could refuse a demanding father or fail to follow medical advice found on an "authoritative, reliable, and accurate" website?

WHY DOCTORS ARE SUED

Doctors are right to worry about being sued. Unfortunately, their worry costs all of us a lot of money.

Patients sue doctors for a variety of reasons. It seems certain, though, that if doctors did not have access to money – insurance, personal, and business assets – few people would sue. There would be no incentive. Instead, doctors who violate laws would go to prison, and those who hurt people would be forced to quit.

The fact is that accidents happen. Accidents happen often. People who suffer as a result of accidents often receive financial reimbursement for temporary or permanent disabilities, and lost wages for time out of work. Some injured persons will bring a lawsuit against those who cause the injury. These kinds of cases are called torts. "Technically, a tort is any civil wrong in which a damaged victim can seek legal redress from the individual who caused the harm..."[3] – lawsuits against doctors, for instance.

During 1950, tort lawsuits for all causes cost U.S. residents about $15 billion (about .6 percent of Gross Domestic Product). Those costs exploded during the next 50 years. "Including insured and self-insured costs, the U.S. tort system cost $233 billion in 2002..." or 2.23 percent of GDP;[4] and it continues to grow faster than the economy.

Of that $233 billion, about $24.6 billion was spent on medical malpractice cases. The price of settling medical

---

3. *Tort Reform*, News Batch, February, 2005.

4. Tillinghast Towers-Perrin, "U.S. Tort Costs: 2003 Update, Trends and Findings on the Costs of the U.S. Tort System."

malpractice cases is growing faster than all other tort costs. Thirty years ago, the total cost of medical malpractice was only $1.2 billion. At 24.6 billion, it means these costs had risen by a staggering 2,000 percent during that time.

WHAT HAPPENED?

Did the spike in malpractice lawsuits happen because medical schools suddenly began graduating incompetent doctors? Are today's doctors just greedy, careless, and distracted by golf? Or was something else going on?

The authors discovered five surprising answers to these questions.

> 1) Tort laws had changed radically during the last 20 years.
> 2) State legislators changed tort laws.
> 3) The law changes created windfall profits for one industry.
> 4) That industry is one of the largest contributors to political campaigns.
> 5) That single industry is so politically powerful that the 1994 health care bill specifically protected their windfall profits.

The underlying reason that the number of medical malpractice lawsuits have spiked, then, is because politics plays favorites. It is one of the strongest arguments against giving the control of your health care to governments.

Moreover, the rising costs associated with malpractice lawsuits contribute directly to the overall increase in health care spending. They do this two ways. First, they increase medical malpractice insurance premiums that all providers must pay, and which they pass on to you in higher fees.

Secondly, they create a climate of fear among doctors that they might lose their license and ability to practice; this drives them to order or prescribe services that protect them against a jury finding them guilty of malpractice.

LAWS CHANGED

About 20 years ago, many states changed their tort laws. Prior to that time, a person "was required to show a complete absence of personal negligence in order to recover [financial damages]."[5] That is, to collect money from someone else, the injured person had to show that they had nothing to do with the cause of their own problem.

Today, many states allow a person to collect damages if they can show that the other party had more to do with their loss than they did. These tort law changes created many more opportunities to sue and win monetary damage awards than had been true before legislators liberalized the laws to favor their friends.

During the time that legislators liberalized tort laws, the number of practicing attorneys increased dramatically, at a rate three times greater than that of the population. About 25 percent of attorneys are involved in representing people who bring personal injury and medical malpractice lawsuits. This type of attorney is usually called a "trial lawyer" or "plaintiff's attorney."

For the average person, bringing a lawsuit, however, means overcoming a major barrier: Trial lawyers are very expensive, and the average-income person cannot afford their fees.

To make their services affordable, trial lawyers take most tort cases on a contingency fee payment arrangement. This means that the attorneys pay and risk all the costs of

---

5. See note 3.

the lawsuit, and are not paid anything until and unless there is a financial settlement. When their client prevails, and money is paid from the other party to them, the trial lawyers collect a fee that is usually 33.3 percent of the financial settlement, plus their expenses. Estimates vary, but "...it has been estimated that claimants [i.e., the person with the injury] ultimately collect only 46 percent of the total cost of the tort system."[6] This is what has created windfall profits for trial lawyers.

Here is an example:

> In an August 2005 settlement of a case against the Merck company, a Texas jury awarded the Robert Ernst family $253 million. The jury had decided that Vioxx contributed to Mr. Ernst's death – he was 59 years old, about six years from retirement. "The jury broke down the damage award as $450,000 in economic damages – Robert Ernst's lost pay as a Wal-Mart produce manager; $24 million for mental anguish and loss of companionship, and $229 million in punitive damages."[7]
>
> The more conservative Texas legislature, however, had put a cap on punitive damages (a punitive damage is like a fine). The final Ernst award will more likely be about $26 million. At this, the trial lawyers will still make more than $8.6 million in legal fees – plus expenses. Had the original damage award prevailed, the attorneys stood to make $83.5 million. No doctor makes this kind of money in such a short period of time.

6. Ibid.
7. MoreLaw.com, "A Litigation Digest & Directory," http://www.morelaw.com/verdicts/case.asp?n=Unknown&s=TX%20%20%20%20%20%20%20&d=30443

WHY DOES THIS GO ON?

Trial lawyers give a lot of money to political campaigns. In fact, between 1989 and 2004, the American Trial Lawyers Association (ATLA) ranks the third largest among direct donors to federal election campaigns (the American Medical Association doctors ranked eleventh). In soft money contributions, ATLA lawyers gave 78 times as much as doctors during 2002.[8] [9] More than 90 percent of ATLA contributions go to Democrats, while the AMA favors Republicans at 80 percent.

So, the same trial lawyers who contribute such large sums of money to politicians, also profit from liberalized tort laws. Their friendship with lawmakers makes it more difficult to win necessary law changes that would help reduce the spiraling cost of health care.

Furthermore, trial lawyers received special protection in the 1994 health care bill, the one that would have created a national health care system. The bill included language that made sure that trial lawyers would be able to continue receiving their contingency fees (windfall profits) at 33.3 percent.[10] No such language existed to protect the fees of any health care provider. On the contrary, federal Medicare law has put tight limits on what providers are paid, and if they try to charge more, they can lose their right to treat Medicare patients. This is a great example of how some politicians favor their friends.

SUING THE DOCTOR CAUSES ILLS

To protect themselves against the costs of a lawsuit,

8. Opensecrets.org, "Top All-Time Donor Profiles," http://www.opensecrets.org/
9. Ibid., "Soft money for lawyers and lobbyists," 2000.
10. H.R. 3600, 103rd Congress, 1994, lines 1-10, 944.

providers buy medical malpractice insurance. As liberal tort laws spurred on more lawsuits, the financial losses of the malpractice insurance companies became staggering. "[Medical malpractice] underwriting losses exploded by $2.7 billion or 938% between 1996 and 2001."[11] The St. Paul Companies, the largest medical malpractice insurance company at the time, quit writing that insurance after 2001. Others followed suit, while still others just continued to raise the premiums.

The effects of increased malpractice insurance premiums is that your health care costs go up and some doctors quit practicing. OB-GYN doctors have, in some places, quit delivering babies – more than 18 percent of Pennsylvanian and 20 percent of West Virginian OB-GYN doctors.

Insurance costs for OB-GYN doctors are three times that of the average for all doctors. Trial lawyers know that when a medical procedure includes delivery of a baby and something goes wrong, juries respond to their emotional pleas and the mental state of their distressed client. That is why OB-GYN doctors pay so much more for medical malpractice insurance. This also drives up the cost of delivering a baby.

In fact, a 2002 study showed that the number one worry of doctors is malpractice lawsuits. They worry about increased insurance costs, but also about professional standing and the time and agony of going through a trial.

So They Go on the Defensive

The threat of a malpractice lawsuit affects the way doctors practice medicine. "That fear of litigation has also caused many to practice defensive medicine, which in turn increases health care costs. Nearly four out of five doctors

---

11. "Medical Malpractice Insurance," Insurance Information Institute, June, 2003, 13.

(79 percent) surveyed said they have ordered unnecessary tests, while 74 percent have referred patients to specialists more often than they would have based solely on professional judgment."[12]

The U.S. Department of Health and Human Services "...suggests that health care costs could be reduced by 5 percent to 9 percent if unreasonable awards for non-economic damages were limited. It estimates this would save $60 billion to $108 billion in health care costs each year..."[13]

Given that "[a]bout 50 percent of health care spending is eaten up by waste, excessive prices and fraud,"[14] it is certain that some portion of this margin of waste results from too much defensive doctoring.

The fear that doctors exhibit about lawsuits have other serious implications that can directly affect you. If, as a result of malpractice costs and concerns, a large number of doctors quit practicing medicine, and if smaller hospitals and health clinics shut down, you might find yourself without help when a tragedy hits. That, of course, is the ultimate cost.

SOME OTHER SIDE EFFECTS OF MEDICAL LAWSUITS

Other issues arise out of medical malpractice lawsuits, and they threaten access to health care and directly drive up its costs.

Each time a doctor is sued and the public learns about it, respect for the medical profession diminishes. Patients trust doctors less. Doctors trust patients less. When people

---

12. Ibid., 5.

13. Ibid., 6.

14. Alan Sager and Deborah Socolar, "Health Costs Absorb One-Quarter of Economic Growth, 2000-2005," Boston University.

begin to mistrust doctors, they also become more sensitive to faultfinding. They look for mistakes and sometimes see them where they do not exist.

When all the medical lawsuits and settlements are added up, along with the additional expense of defensive medicine, these costs must be paid by someone. Insurance companies, HMOs, and governments write the checks, but they get their money through premiums and taxes. Doctors pay the medical malpractice insurance premiums, but have to add those costs to what they charge you.

No one believes that medical providers should be shielded from lawsuits. Doctors who hurt people should pay for the damage. A justice system that strikes a balance between patients' and doctors' needs is a reasonable answer. This is difficult to do since each of the 50 states write their own tort laws. Malpractice lawsuits are far more common in some states than others, because those states have made it easier to sue and recover damages. Many believe that the federal government must step in and solve this problem by establishing tort laws that are the same in all 50 states.

We all have a great stake in reforming the tort system in a way that removes the fear and overwhelming expense from doctors, and that provides a financial remedy when accidents occur.

The current tort system has been tried and found guilty of increasing your cost of health care.

CHAPTER 7
PAYING THE BILLS: HEALTH INSURANCE & "FREE HEALTH CARE"

During 2003, we Americans spent $1.7 trillion on health care.[1] That is a lot of money, and hard to imagine. So who pays out all this money?

There are two types of health care payers: government and non-government (private sector).

The government pays for health care through Medicare, Medicaid, and dozens of other programs. You can read about them in chapters eight and nine. Government programs pay for the health care of 77 million people (26 percent of U.S. residents). The cost of providing health care to this group was $766 billion in 2003 – 46 percent of health care spending.[2] These government-paid health care programs spent $9,948 per person ($766 billion divided by 77 million).

Non-government health care is paid for by insurance companies, HMOs and private persons. Non-government spending on health care totaled 54 percent of the total, or about $930 billion. That is an average of about $4,285 per

---

1 "Table 1, National Health Expenditures Aggregate and per Capita Amounts, Percent Distribution, and Average Annual Percent Growth, by Source of Funds: Selected Calendar Years 1980-2003," Center for Medicare and Medicaid Services, United States Government.
2 Ibid.

person. This is less than half of what the government spends per person ($930 billion divided by 217 million). Another way of saying this is that government spends more than twice as much per person for health care than does the private sector.

About 60 percent of U.S. residents have some or all of their health insurance paid for by their employers, while about nine percent pay for their own insurance.[3]

(The federal government reports that governments pay the insurance costs of 26 percent of Americans, employers pay for 60 percent, and private parties pay for 9 percent, for a total of 95 percent. This presents a curious dilemma for health care reformers, because it means that 5 percent are, presumably, uninsured. Yet health care reformers report that more than 15 percent of U.S. residents are uninsured. *Be sure to read chapter 13 on the uninsured issue.*)

A BRIEF HISTORY OF U.S. HEALTH INSURANCE

All types of insurance operate on the principle of shared risk. You pay premiums to an insurance company, and the company uses your premiums to pay claims. You purchase insurance on your life, home, automobile, collector's items, businesses, health; there are dozens of kinds of insurance.

When you purchase auto insurance, you hope never to use it. Only when the unexpected happens – an accident, storm damage, theft, vandalism – do you file a claim. You would never expect your insurance to pay for regular auto maintenance such as an oil change, tire rotation, or a tune-up. Until the mid-1960s, Americans looked at their health insurance in the same way: they expected to use it only to

---

3. "Historical Health Insurance Tables, Table HI-1. Health Insurance Coverage Status and Type of Coverage by Sex, Race and Hispanic Origin: 1987-2003," http://www.census.gov/hhs/www/hlthins/historic/hihistt.html

help pay the costs of unexpected catastrophic illness or injury, not preventive care. That is why it was called catastrophic or major medical insurance.

Insurance companies make their policies affordable by offering similar coverage to a large number of people, and collecting premiums from all of them. Premiums collected from everyone pay the costs of those needing care, and the insurance company's operating costs. The insurance policy specifies which health care services are covered. Insured persons who want to purchase health care services not covered by their insurance policy are free to do so, but they must pay those costs themselves, without insurance company reimbursement.

In the United States, employer-provided health insurance began in the 1940s, but some companies had made it available much earlier than that.

"In the 1870s...railroad, mining, and other industries began to provide the services of company doctors to workers. In 1910, Montgomery Ward entered into one of the earliest group insurance contracts."[4] At the turn of the twentieth century, the Hershey Company sweetened their employees' lives by providing company doctors and hospitals. Essentially, however, no one had health insurance in the United States until the 1920s, when Blue Cross first offered hospitalization insurance.

During the 1940s, Blue Shield also began offering a limited form of insurance for payments to doctors and other non-hospital health care providers. Both Blue Cross and Blue Shield only paid for catastrophic health care costs. Individuals paid for the bulk of their own health care. They went to the doctor of their choice, and with the doctor's advice, made decisions about which treatments to pursue; then they paid their doctor.

---

4. Facts from EBRI, "History of Health Insurance Benefits," March 2002, http://www.ebri.org/facts/0302fact.htm

During the 1940s as World War II raged, the federal government placed wage controls on employers. This meant that they could not give wage increases to workers. The government did, however, make health insurance an option for employers to help retain their best workers, and attract new ones. The federal government said that neither workers nor employers would have to pay any kind of taxes on employer-paid health insurance premiums. That law remains in effect today, and has been recently extended to include self-employed people.

FROM ENVELOPES TO ENTITLEMENTS

Until the mid-1960s, Americans paid for as much as 47 percent of their own health care out of their own pocket.[5] If they owned insurance, it only covered major expenses that protected them from unforeseen catastrophic medical and hospital bills.

People paid a fee each time they used a doctor or hospital – called a fee-for-service. Most people who owned health insurance expected that they might need it a handful of times during their lifetime – hopefully, never.

Many families kept an envelope at home in which they stored their medical receipts for the bills they had paid. If they filled the envelope with enough receipts, and their expenses exceeded their deductible, they submitted a claim to their insurance company. They seldom exceeded their deductible.

Paying for a medical service was the same as paying someone to fix a transmission, remodel a room, or install a new carpet. In this way, millions of Americans making independent purchasing decisions each day pumped tens of

---

5. "National Health Expenditures by Type of Service & Source of Funds: Calendar Years 1960-2004," Centers for Medicaid & Medicare, U.S. Government, 3.

millions of dollars into the health care economy. As medical service providers watched how people spent their health care dollars, they knew what services they should offer. These services were further augmented by breakthroughs in medical technology and procedures. Free markets work this way, finding solutions to problems that purchasers want solved.

Families had a close personal relationship with a general practitioner. Since they paid their own medical bills, health care lined up against all the other family purchasing decisions, and sometimes that meant not calling the doctor unless someone was quite ill. Doctors' fees had to be affordable so that people would have the funds to pay for their services. Often, doctors made house calls; and why not, since the family directly paid their bills. The doctor had a direct interest in keeping patients happy.

During the early 1960s, about six percent of U.S. residents were older than 64, and only half of those owned health insurance. Congress used that 50 percent uninsured rate as reason to create a new, centralized payment system for the health care needs of seniors. In 1965, Congress created Medicare to provide hospital and doctor services to seniors aged 65 and older.

Also in 1965, Congress created Medicaid, a taxpayer-paid insurance program for low-income, and some disabled and aged Americans. Before this, doctors often provided free care to low-income persons, and they sent them to the county hospital for severe illness or injury. Scores of charities, often faith-based, provided medical care for indigents and low-income people.

The next two chapters discuss Medicare, Medicaid and other government health care programs in depth. Here we refer to them only to demonstrate the change in the mindset of health care consumers tied directly to these government programs.

As a result of Medicare and Medicaid, for the first time in United States' history, some Americans discovered they were entitled to nearly free coverage for a wide range of health care services. These benefits, however, exceeded those available to the vast majority of 1965 U.S. workers whose insurance only covered catastrophic illness or disease. U.S. seniors and low-income residents could now throw away the receipt envelope and sign up for a fantastic, and nearly free, health care entitlement. Government now paid for most of their health care and patients had no clue about its costs; neither did they much care, since someone else paid the bills.

For those Medicare and Medicaid patients, health care providers (i.e., doctors, hospitals, clinics) now received their reimbursements directly from the government. The government quickly realized that it needed to control overall costs. They directed that effort at providers. Providers saw their payment levels drop, and struggled to keep up with inflation as the government began limiting those reimbursements. To keep up financially, doctors had to see more patients, cutting down on the time spent with each.

Now that they were entitled to nearly free health care, Medicare and Medicaid patients increased their utilization of medical services – they demanded care more often. In 1965, the government spent $10.6 billion on health care; but that had ballooned to $28.3 billion by 1970,[6] increasing at a rate nearly twice as fast as privately paid health care.[7] Health care spending worried the lawmakers who created the programs. Acting in the manner of politicians, to solve this funding problem, Congress decided to pass more laws.

---

6. Ibid., 2-3.
7. "No. 114. National Health Expenditures–Summary, 1960-2002, and Projections, 2003-2013," Abstract of the United States, Bureau of the Census.

THE CYCLE: FROM INSURANCE TO ENTITLEMENTS

Myth: Health care had become such a problem that the U.S. government had to get involved.

Truth: When the government tries to solve a problem, it creates new problems that eventually it also tries to solve, creating an endless cycle of problem-solving.

During the late 1960s, the Nixon Administration fretted about the future explosion of health care costs, as seniors and low-income people had already begun taking advantage of nearly unlimited free health care from Medicare and Medicaid. Congress had also witnessed health care costs increase at an average of 13.3 percent for those with private insurance from 1970 to 1973.[8] They believed they needed a new management model to slow down the spiraling cost increases. In 1973, Congress passed legislation to create the Health Maintenance Organization (HMO), and it radically changed the nature of the delivery of health care for everyone from insurance-based to one of entitlement.

Those 1970s health care reformers believed that the HMO could save money and increase the quality of health care. Congress' goal was to do for those aged 64 and younger what it had done for those aged 65 and older who were now on Medicare – entitle them to a wide range of health care services.

Unlike fee-for-service insurance that paid a provider only after they provided a service, HMOs offered *pre-paid* health care services. They called this "capitation." "Capitation means that the provider is paid a certain amount of dollars per member in the HMO. This payment is made to

---

8. "Table 12: Per Enrollee Expenditures and Growth in Medicare Spending and Private Health Insurance Premiums, Calendar Years 1969-2003," Centers for Medicare and Medicaid Services, United States.

the provider whether they see the members or not."[9] Each month, the HMO received a premium payment, whether or not the insured person used medical services. From the pay-as-you-go system under catastrophic insurance, HMOs offered a pay-before-you-go system.

HMO leaders believed that they could reduce overall health care spending in the long run by providing preventive care services. Keeping healthy people healthy, and nipping sickness in the bud, they reasoned, would fight off high costs in the decades that followed.

A noticeable shift in patient attitude soon followed, and it paralleled what had happened with Medicare and Medicaid. A person's mindset under fee-for-service had been, "Okay, do we really need to see the doctor for that sore throat? I only have $52 in my checking account." As an HMO member, that attitude became, "Hey, why not go to the doctor? We already pre-paid for the service anyway." Patients now felt entitled to see the doctor because their employer had pre-paid the HMO.

THE LOCKED GATE

The first HMOs were called "closed-ended, staff" models. This meant that persons who purchased HMO services were limited to using only the doctors who were HMO employees. (Before this, patients could go to any doctor and for any purpose, as long as they paid the bill. Doctors had been self-employed or in a partnership, working in fee-for-service practices that they usually owned.)

Those early HMO models that the government designed in the 1973 HMO act, used a primary care gatekeeper doctor. The gatekeeper doctor strictly controlled the patient's ability to receive additional health care services.

9. "Health Care Cost, HMOs, PPOs, EPOs,"
http://members.tripod.com/proagency/insurance0.html

They especially controlled access to diagnostic tests and specialists. This type of HMO looked like this:

> As you stand talking to the primary care doctor, you glance behind him and see a gate. On the other side of that gate you see a lineup of medical specialists who may have been more qualified to treat your condition than the primary care doctor. You like your doctor, but when you ask him to open the gate and let you see a specialist, he refuses.
>
> The doctor explains that it is not medically necessary for you to see a specialist. He does not tell you that the HMO business administrator would discipline him if he opened the gate, nor does he tell you that if he let you go to a specialist, his clinic would have to pay that specialist's fee, not your insurance company (and in some HMO models, it cost the doctor personally).
>
> You went to the doctor because you thought your child had strep throat. The doctor looked at your child and recommended Tylenol and bed rest. The doctor refused to take a throat culture until your third visit, hoping that the sore throat would disappear, and at the same time, saving the clinic the cost of a diagnostic test. The doctor did this because the administrator had imposed a strict practice guideline on him.
>
> The doctor valued his job and, at the same time, wanted to do right by you. You, however, believed that your health care benefit allowed you free access to specialists and

diagnostic tests, if ever you had a need. A conflict developed between the gatekeeper doctor
and you, and you blamed him.

HMOs gave doctors the financial incentive to keep you
healthy. They did this by intervening with preventive care,
so that you would enjoy better health for a lifetime. Keeping you healthy would reduce the number of times you
needed to see a doctor, and it would save money on medical expenses. Since the HMO doctor received the same
monthly payment no matter whether you ever came to see
him, or came 10 times a month, it was to his advantage to
keep you healthy. The less often you came, the more he
could earn.

Too often, patients came to label the gatekeeper doctor
as the "bad guy." The patient liked the entitlement to see a
doctor anytime they wished, but resented the gatekeeper
who kept them from the care they wanted.

Even today, it's a common plot line in TV serials about
the practice of medicine. The popular show "ER" frequently has an element in which the emergency room doctor is
told to "discharge, discharge, discharge," even when the
doctor believes that patient needs more treatment. Controlling costs, it seemed, became more important than curing
disease.

If a patient demanded to go to a doctor outside of the
old, closed-ended HMO, the patient paid for it, and this
created resentments.

HMO managers had optimistically set their premiums
low to attract large employer groups. The federal government further reduced HMO premiums with a $375 million
subsidy.[10] That subsidy was not available to companies that
wrote traditional catastrophic fee-for-service insurance,

---

10. William Wenmark, "Minnesota Health Care Marketplace Reform," 2005.

giving HMOs a competitive advantage, paid for by federal taxes.

Furthermore, to encourage large groups to join, the federal government mandated that all large employers had to offer HMOs as an option to their employees, if an HMO operated in their area. Naturally, workers often opted for the HMO because it offered more benefits at a lower cost.

A DIFFERENT WAY OF PAYING THE DOCTOR BILL

Many Americans decided that the closed-ended, staff HMO with its gatekeeper doctor was far too rigid, so HMOs adapted. Some, while still employing their own doctors, allowed the patient to seek care outside of the HMO. In such cases, the HMO had to pay the non-HMO doctor out of the monthly premium it collected from the employer. They resisted sending patients outside of their HMO.

Some doctors, who refused to be employed by HMOs, still wanted the income from seeing HMO patients. Many formed independent partnerships, and those partnerships contracted with the HMOs to handle some of the patient load.

HMOs have since created Preferred Provider Organizations (PPOs) to broaden their benefits. In a PPO, the HMO negotiates reimbursements with a wide assortment of doctors, clinics, and hospitals to provide care for its members. This is the most popular HMO model today.

OLDER DOCTORS RESISTED

At the beginning, HMOs faced several critical problems, not the least of which was to change the ingrained habits of doctors and their patients. Patients with long-standing ties to a doctor wanted to keep seeing the same doctor, but could not. Instead, they had to see an HMO-employed doctor if they wanted the plan to pay the doctor's bill. As well, HMOs had a tough time getting older, more experienced doctors to work for them.

Experienced doctors had been used to making all their own treatment decisions. In an HMO (and later, in other forms of managed care) doctors were forced to follow strict practice guidelines monitored by an HMO nurse or other HMO employee.

Managed care turned to yet another kind of group, called a Utilization Review Organization (URO), to step in to review and establish best practice guidelines – some labeled this "cookie cutter medicine." Such an arrangement frustrated both the more established doctors and their patients, and patients often did not understand – so they blamed the doctors.

To hire doctors, then, the earliest HMOs looked to younger physicians, many of whom had just finished their medical residency or internship. The HMOs offered these young doctors stable hours, – often 40-50 hours per week, just like other professionals – an excellent salary, modern equipment, assured patient load, and none of the frustrations of running a private practice. These young doctors did not offer as much resistance to managed care as did older, experienced doctors.

A good number of those young doctors really *were* able to deliver a better level of care, unshackled by outmoded delivery systems, and less-than-informed habits. Some of the established doctors, though they resented the imposition of discipline from managed care, admitted that it provided them with efficiencies that they sorely needed.

Many doctors would not consider themselves to be great business managers, and they preferred just to practice medicine. HMOs helped organize their practice, and provided business management services.

The explosion of technology and medical break-throughs during this time further complicated the practice of medicine, and HMOs and other forms of managed care helped the doctor take advantage of these changes. So HMOs, especially to older doctors, became a love-hate relationship – they resented having to get permission to practice, but appreciated the management help they got in return.

SELLING HMO PLANS

Selling HMO plans was easy. The HMO marketers and insurance agents who sold them highlighted several advantages for their prospective clients.

HMO plans emphasized preventive health care, thus directly appealing to young, healthy families. Some of these families had previously forgone health insurance because, given their good health, they felt no need for it, unless their employer offered it to them. If they did have employer coverage, they were high deductible plans – $100. Typically, they only saw a doctor when someone became quite ill.

HMOs offered expanded benefits, like the chance to get regular physicals and immunizations for their children at no extra cost. Mothers really liked being able to take their children to the doctor anytime they had a fever, sore throat or cough – some even threw away their thermometers, knowing they could always go to the doctor to have a child's temperature taken. Since the services were pre-paid, families felt entitled to use them.

Single people, especially young ones, often chose not to own health insurance. Affordable HMOs, though, with their emphasis on preventive care, appealed to them.

The early HMOs wrote plans without requiring any underwriting (known as guaranteed issue), meaning that a person's health history played no role in whether they would be covered under the health plan. This was a dramatic change from how fee-for-service plans worked. Fee-for-service plans had to anticipate projected costs, and to do so meant knowing the health history of those who were insured. Sicker people require more services and, therefore are more expensive to insure. Fee-for-service insurers set their rates higher for less healthy individuals and groups.

HMOs had one set rate based on the benefits offered, and ignored individual and group health history. Because of guaranteed issue, a person could wait until they became ill before choosing an HMO plan during open enrollment (the time at which they were given the chance to choose a new plan for the next year). Insurance agents could move entire groups of less healthy people to HMOs where they could get more benefits at a lower rate. These less healthy groups created a great deal of tension between administrators, gatekeeper doctors, and patients, as HMOs fought to keep per-patient costs in line. They also shocked some HMO doctors who had believed they would be caring mostly for healthy patients.

Younger families and singles had not yet established a long-term relationship with a doctor, so it was easy for them to accept the idea that, at the clinic, they might see a different doctor each time. What became hard for them, however, was when they became more seriously ill. The gatekeeper doctor did not always give them access to the care they desired.

Costs Went Up

Myth: HMOs would serve the dual purpose of controlling health care costs and keeping people healthier.

Truth: HMOs encouraged more utilization and health care spending went up.

Truth: When the government intervened in private health care, spending accelerated.

Congress believed that the gatekeeper doctor in an HMO would control overall health care spending. Instead, health care costs rose dramatically.

During the 10 years following the creation of HMOs, Medicare health care spending went up an average of 15.8 percent a year, while those with private insurance and pre-paid HMO plans saw their spending increase 15.3 percent a year.[11]

From 1974-1983, general inflation averaged 8.5 percent per year.[12] That meant that health care spending increases nearly doubled that of other consumer prices. A $100 non-health care purchase in 1974 had grown to $202 by 1983. Medicare spending, however, had gone from $568 per enrollee in 1974, to $2,027 by 1984,[13] when it should have grown to about $1,148. Private spending on health care, despite the federal government's authorization of HMOs, rose from $161 to $596 during the same period, instead of the $284 that would have tracked general inflation.[14]

How the patient viewed health care had also changed dramatically during those 10 years. From the 1960s, when most people expected to use health insurance a few times during their life – or maybe never – Americans began to use health care a few times a year, or more.

---

11. See note 8.
12. http://www.minneapolisfed.org/Research/data/us/calc/hist1913.cfm
13. See note 8.
14. Ibid.

Americans had come to view health insurance as an entitlement, and claimed the right to go to the doctor as often as they wished, *because someone else paid the bill.*

HMOs changed the doctor-patient relationship as well. Prior to HMOs, when the patient had paid directly for his or her own health care, they usually had a healthy respect for, and were loyal to one doctor. With HMOs, the patient may have seen a different doctor during each visit, and they had no control over which doctor they got to see. The doctor they saw acted as their gatekeeper, and if the patient did not like one doctor's answer, they would try to see someone else. This lack of a personal doctor-patient relationship came to create tension and mistrust between many patients and their doctors.

As HMOs came to be the preferred choice of large employer groups, traditional fee-for-service insurance plans nearly died out completely. They could hardly compete in big cities where the HMOs flourished, and had to go to the rural areas and small towns, where HMOs had a tough time finding enough patients to make a system work.

Patients who had chronic health problems and a choice of health plans eventually left the old HMOs, desiring more control over their care. They went back to fee-for-service plans to avoid the gatekeeper. This was more like the traditional doctor-patient relationship. Traditional insurance companies, however, saw their costs increase as they attracted less healthy persons (called adverse selection). These insurance companies lost a lot of business to HMOs: especially that of healthier persons. The business they managed to retain cost them more, while competitive pressures forced them to offer more benefits, such as preventive care, cancer screenings, and such. Many traditional fee-for-service insurance companies quit the business.

Small employers and individuals, too, found it increasingly difficult to purchase health insurance. Some went without insurance for a period of time. By the 1980s, health care reformers pointed to reports of a growing number of uninsured persons and called it a "crisis."

Medicare, Medicaid, and low-cost HMOs, all created by Congress, were supposed to keep prices down while raising quality. All three programs, however, suffered from the same problem: patients did not know the cost of care, and neither were they responsible to pay for it. Someone else paid the bills – an entitlement mindset had taken root.

HEALTH CARE
BREAKTHROUGHS INCREASED SPENDING

U.S. ingenuity, fueled by a red-hot 1980s economy, added to health care spending. Drug companies, medical device manufacturers, and medical researchers brought new treatments into the health care marketplace. The payers and politicians heard from health care consumers – they wanted access to those new developments, and they wanted health insurance to pay the bills.

State governments mandated that insurers pay for dozens of new procedures, devices, drugs, treatments, alternative practices, and almost anything else called health care. Though these mandates also increased premiums, legislators pointed out that in the long term, they should save money, and they would reduce pain and suffering.

Some examples:

> Legislators mandated that doctor-deliv-
> ered maternity care must be a fully covered
> benefit, including pre-natal, delivery, and post-
> delivery costs. Cancer victims undergoing
> chemotherapy wanted insurance to pay for
> wigs so that they could maintain their dignity.

Advocates for those who abused drugs and alcohol wanted insurance-paid treatment which they felt sure would save the cost of a liver transplant, or the long-term costs generated by dementia.

As legislators added mandates, the cost of health insurance increased. The strong U.S. economy readily absorbed most of these cost increases, but some people had to drop their health insurance, unable to afford the more expensive premiums.

During the long sustained economic recovery that ran from the mid-1980s to the late 1990s, unemployment remained low. Employers, competing for new hires, continued to sweeten the health care segment of their benefit packages, even though their cost per employee grew higher every year. Sometimes a new job applicant asked about the health benefits even before wanting to know the salary. As well, most union contracts specified 100 percent employer-paid coverage for the best available health insurance or HMO plans.

The cost of traditional insurance policies and HMO plans, now loaded up with numerous types of benefits, began to soar. Employers began shifting more of that expense to employees. The HMOs and insurance companies began requiring patients to pay higher co-payments.

PLANS COST EMPLOYEES MORE

In 1980, requiring employees to pay a small part of their insurance or HMO premiums received very little resistance. Then, employees paid $1 to $5 a week, and up to $10 a week for family coverage.

Paying a little of the cost for access to more services

seemed reasonable. Trading a few dollars of income to be able to get a physical, or see the doctor when they wanted to go, or have some of their prescription costs covered, made sense. By 1995, the individual employee's portion had risen to $15 a week, and about $40 a week for dependents' insurance. Employees noticed, but preferred to maintain or even add benefits to their plans.

People who worked for employers that did not provide health insurance benefits, and self-employed persons, had to buy their own insurance. Healthier people opted for policies with high deductibles – $500-$2,500 – to hold down the cost of a family policy. Families with health problems tried to buy policies with lower deductibles, although they were relatively costly. Insurance companies attached riders to their policies that denied certain benefits to a person with chronic or preexisting health problems.

Some people with health problems purchased their insurance from health risk pools – plans set up by states to insure the "uninsurables." These premiums are usually higher than a regular policy, but as much as 50 percent of its true cost is paid by an assessment against health insurance companies. This makes it possible for "uninsurable" persons to have a chance to purchase health insurance at an affordable price.

HMOs had mostly become open-ended by the mid-1990s, and had PPOs that allowed enrollees to go outside their networks. In many ways, they looked more like fee-for-service plans and nothing like the original, rigid closed-ended, staff gatekeeper plans that Congress had intended.

By 1993, health care costs had soared to 13.3 percent of the Gross Domestic Product.[15] The U.S. Census Bureau announced that the uninsured rate had grown to nearly 14 percent.[16] Reformers declared we had *another* health care

15. See note 1.
16. Table No. 139, Statistical abstract of the United States, 2003, Bureau of the Census.

"crisis." This is what caused First Lady Hillary Clinton to call together her health care study group in Washington, D.C. They planned to finally solve the crisis.

The Clinton plan relied on the federal government to control health care, in a sense in the way it had hoped HMO administrators would have acted. By their votes in the 1994 election, Americans strongly and directly rejected the Clinton plan. We were unwilling to hand over one-seventh of the economy to government managers.

HEALTH CARE CONSUMER PROTECTION

Myth: Health care providers and insurance companies created unbearable tension between them and their patients, and it required government to step in to referee.

Truth: Government intrusion into private health care created the tension between patients, providers, and payers, through the HMO gatekeeper system.

The tension and mistrust between patients, providers, and payers escalated. In 1996, President Bill Clinton issued an Executive Order to create a commission which he charged to "...advise the President on changes occurring in the health care system and, where appropriate, to make recommendations on how best to promote and assure consumer protection and health care quality."[17]

During the 1997 budget debates, Congress began to consider passing a Patients' Bill of Rights. By so doing, Congress finally admitted it had failed in 1973. Instead of creating a health care system that would control costs and improve quality, the 1973 law had increased utilization by creating entitlement thinking; spending went up dramatically. Though the quality of health care had continued to improve, patients came to mistrust doctors; doctors felt

---

17. "President's Advisory Commission on Consumer Protection and Quality in the Health Care Industry," the charter. http://www.hcqualitycommission.gov/charter.html

cheated by payers (insurance companies, HMOs, and the government); and payers were besieged by consumers who demanded more benefits.

During March of 1998, President Clinton's health care commission issued its final report. It contained dozens of recommendations, chief among them was the right for "...direct access to a qualified specialist of their choice within a plan's network of providers."[18] Patients wanted the gatekeeper to open the gate.

Since then, most payers and providers have adopted some form of a Patient's Bill of Rights, and a printed form of these are available for the asking. Common to them is a patient's "...right to a choice of health care providers that is sufficient to ensure access to appropriate high-quality health care."[19] Such statements may not carry the force of law, but they do give patients basis to sue if they are denied care according to the listed rights.

In 2002, the U.S. Senate passed the McCain-Edwards-Kennedy Patients' Bill of Rights, but the House did not concur and the law failed. The 2002 Senate bill would have ensured that patients had the right to:

- have their medical decisions made by a doctor;
- see a medical specialist;
- go to the closest emergency room;
- designate a pediatrician as a primary care doctor for their children;
- keep the same doctor throughout their medical treatment;
- obtain the prescription drugs their doctor prescribes;

18 Ibid. Chapter Two, "Choice of Providers and Plans." http://hcqualitycommission.gov/cborr/chap2.html
19 Ibid.

> ◆ access a fair and independent
> appeals process if care is denied;
> ◆ hold their health plan accountable for
> harm done.[20]

Still today, Congress continues to try to fix this thorny problem through national legislation. Perhaps it is trying to turn back the clock to the days before it created Medicare, Medicaid, and HMOs, when patients were in control because they knew the price of health care, since they paid their own bills.

HEALTH INSURANCE ADAPTED, AGAIN

The honeymoon of free entitlement health care enjoyed by employers and employees started to come to an end by 2000. The delusion that Americans could receive unlimited care at others' expense – something for nothing – finally hit home. Years of added benefits, spiraling health care costs, and insurance premiums, had been offset by general prosperity. Low unemployment rates had forced companies to maintain rich health benefit plans. Even though deductibles and co-payments had gone up, wage and salary increases had offset the increased cost.

A recession that began during the fall of 2000 was made worse by the 9-11 terrorist attacks of 2001. As the economy stuttered and then retooled, employers stepped up their efforts to shift more of the cost of health insurance to their employees. Rising unemployment added to the pressure felt by workers to accept reduced health benefits and increased co-pays and deductibles.

By 2003, that 1980s $1-$5 employee weekly cost for single coverage had grown to $10-$40. For a family, the

20. "President's Advisory Commission on Health Care Reform: Consumer Bill of Rights," Chapter Two, Health Care Quality Commission, 1998.

weekly payroll deduction had exploded to $50, or even as much as $250. Co-pays, which had been $2 in the 1980s, became $10, $20, and $30. Everyone noticed, and no one liked it.

The culprit that had driven these higher costs was the idea that someone else pays your health care bills.

Those health care costs are included in the price of all the goods and services that you purchase. For example, "GM...spends $1,500 on health care for each car produced in the United States."[21] So, General Motors must add $1,500 to each car it builds to pay the health insurance costs of the GM employees who build it. It has made their cars less competitively priced and cut into their profits. GM has been providing their employees with 100 percent coverage for a broad range of benefits for decades, and the union has resisted the idea that workers should share in the cost of this benefit. As a result, during November 2005, GM announced the layoff of 30,000 employees. Entitlement thinking threatens GM's ability to stay in business.

By 2002, across the country, the employers' share of the health insurance premium was $3,740 per employee for health care benefits.[22] At this rate, a company with 50 employees spent $187,000 during 2002 to provide a health care benefit. Another company, with 1,000 employees, spent $3.7 million. Health insurance had become very expensive – a major expense.

POLITICIANS DON'T WANT TO SOLVE THIS PROBLEM

Myth: Politicians really want to solve the health care spending problem.

Truth: Politicians use the health care spending problem

---

21 Amy Joyce, "GM's UAW Retirees Face Health Care Costs, Deal Would End Free Coverage," *The Washington Post,* Oct. 21, 2005, D01.
22 The 2002 Employer Benefits Study, U.S. Chamber of Commerce, 2002.

to accumulate more power and influence, and win more votes.

Prominent politicians have made health care reform their centerpiece. They are supported by influence groups who also want to have a voice in the reform debate. Few of them really want to bring down costs, nor do they want to give you back control over your health care decisions.

Many of these national figures believe that every American is entitled to "free" health care, with the government paying the cost. It is the same idea that many 1960s leaders had about Medicare and Medicaid. So they advocate moving to a single-payer health care system, perhaps like Health Canada (see the section on foreign health care, chapters 14-20). Or, they want to mandate that everyone must own health insurance, and look to employers to pay the cost. Mostly, they complain about insurance companies, the pharmaceutical industry, miserly employers, blaming everyone except themselves. Many politicians believe it is good for government to control your health; after all, it gives them more power and influence.

CYCLING DOWN AND CYCLING Up

In the United States, we have learned important lessons since the creation of the entitlement mentality that began with Medicare and Medicaid, and continued with the early HMO models.

The perception of free care increased utilization, sending people to the doctor for less important conditions, putting financial stress on the system, that made it more difficult when the system needed to deal with serious medical problems.

The doctor-patient relationship that had

been one of trust and respect was greatly damaged by the rigid gatekeeper doctor system; by a system of health care that is payer-centered, rather than patient-centered.

Employers and employees are comfortable with the idea of health insurance that is provided by employers, as long as they can afford their share of the premium.

If it is a goal of the health care system to control and even reduce the cost of health care, patients must be involved in the purchasing decision: they must have money at stake to validate their decisions. As it is today, patients have no clue about the cost of even a simple doctor visit, and if they do know, it makes no difference, since someone else pays the bill.

Congress' belief in a centralized effort of cost-containment not only created ill will, but also drove the cost of care higher.

The free market looked back at what had worked before, and is now reacting by once again, putting patients in control of their own health care decisions, as employers move toward insurance policies with higher deductibles.

Americans are a resilient and creative people. We like the idea of shared risk, and private health insurance to pay the bulk of our health care costs. We want the right to choose. We prefer to try to find ways for private sector insurance to pay for health care services.

Medicare and Medicaid, the primary programs for government-paid health care, have been with us since 1965, but few people understand how they work and are funded. Since they fund 46 percent of health care spending, we now turn our attention to these government-gatekeeper systems. They are going in the opposite direction of private health insurance.

CHAPTER 8
MEDICARE
HEALTH CARE ENTITLEMENTS BEGIN

Since its inception in 1965, Medicare has delivered needed health care to tens of millions of Americans. Before Congress passed Medicare, at a time when just six percent of the population was aged 65 or older, only half of America's seniors owned health insurance. Those who owned health insurance had catastrophic coverage, with high deductibles, and paid for most of their own care out of their pockets.

The Medicare plan provided seniors with a basic set of health benefits, that did not include prescription drug coverage nor preventive care. Medicare recipients chose private supplemental health insurance to close the gaps in coverage not provided by Medicare: known as Medigap insurance, or Medicare supplemental insurance. Individuals paid their own premiums for Medigap coverage. When the individual owned a Medigap policy, combined with Medicare, they received greater than 95 percent coverage for hospital and doctor expenses.

Since Medicare and the Medigap policy paid nearly all of a person's health care bills, it gave enrollees the sense that they were entitled to use health services more often than before Medicare. The real costs of health care had become hidden from them, because the government and insurance companies paid most of the bills. Whereas before turning age 65 seniors had to carefully watch each dollar spent on health care, at age 65 they could now use as many services as they felt they needed, and the insurance only cost a few dollars a week.

This marked a dramatic change in the American mindset from self-reliance to dependence on government for one of the most critical of human needs - health. Health is, after all, King of the Hill, the Primary Objective; and now, people looked to the federal government to provide it. Today, more than 40 million U.S. residents subscribe to Medicare.[1] (In 2003, Medicare spent $7,061 per enrollee for health care, compared to $3,088 for persons with private health insurance.[2])

Now when you turn age 65, a surprise awaits you: *Your health care insurance premiums actually go down*, even though you will use health care services far more often than when you were younger. In fact, once you turn 65, your health care insurance premium can drop as much as 70 percent! How is it possible?

The Medicare program today, when combined with Medigap insurance, reduces total out-of-pocket costs to zero for most injuries and illnesses. In 2003, Congress added Part D to cover prescription drug expenses so that a good deal of those costs will also be covered. This combined insurance coverage costs less than $300 a month in most states. A person aged 64 could pay up to $1,000 a month for the same insurance coverage. Just by turning 65,

---

1. "Coverage Center Page," Centers for Medicare and Medicaid Services, United States, http://www.cms.hhs.gov/center/coverage.asp.
2. "Table 12: Per Enrollee Expenditures and Growth in Medicare Spending and Private Health Insurance Premiums, Calendar Years 1969-2003," Centers for Medicare and Medicaid Services, United States.

you may save $700 a month in insurance premiums – 70 percent less than someone aged 64.

How is it possible that costs could drop so much just because someone turns 65? There are four main reasons:

1. taxes on working people;
2. taxes on employers;
3. federal law; and
4. cost shifting through price controls.

MEDICARE TAXES

Myth: The Medicare taxes that you pay during your working life go into your personal Medicare account, and are used to pay your Medicare expenses when you reach age 65 and beyond.

Truth: The Medicare taxes that you pay during your working life are pooled with all other Medicare taxes, and are used to pay the Medicare expenses of all retirees. Most of the Medicare taxes you paid were spent years ago.

Medicare's expenses are paid by a tax on payrolls. Both employees and employers pay the tax.

At the outset, those taxes seemed very reasonable. Anyone earning an income paid a tax of "35/100 of 1 per cent of a worker's wages," with the taxed income capped at $5,600.[3] (There is no longer a cap on taxable income – taxpayers pay the Medicare tax on 100 percent of their earned income.)

In 1965, the average family had one breadwinner, most often the father. In 1966, the breadwinner earning $4,500 a year began paying $15.75 each year out of his check in Medicare taxes. His employer withheld the tax from the employee's paycheck, but it only amounted to about 30

---

3. Honorable Morris Udahl, D-Arizona, "Congressman's Report," March 31, 1965.

cents a week – hardly noticeable. The employer paid the same amount as the employee, for an annual Medicare tax of $31.50 for that worker.

By 1986, that early low tax rate had increased more than 400 percent to 1.45 percent for the employee and the same for the employer, for a total of 2.9 percent. All earned income is now subject to the Medicare tax. Average family income in 2004 had grown to $44,389.[4] This means that the total Medicare tax paid by a modern family and its employers is now $1,287, compared with $31.50 in 1965.

Myth: Forty years experience with Medicare has shown us the government has proven that it can control the upward spiral of health care spending.

Truth: Since the government has not been able to control Medicare spending, payroll taxes have had to increase four times faster than inflation to fund Medicare health spending.

The 1965 breadwinner who earned $4,500 would be earning about $27,500 today, if his pay had just kept even with inflation. The Medicare tax paid by him and his employer, however, would have increased from $31.50 to $798. If Medicare taxes had just tracked general inflation, the 2005 tax should have been $193. The Medicare tax rate had increased more than four times faster than inflation.

Moms and dads of those 1960s teenagers are now in their 80s or 90s, and are receiving benefits far in excess of the taxes they paid during their working lives. The increased costs are being paid by their children, grandchildren, and great-grandchildren.

---

4. "Median Income of Households by Selected Characteristics, 2004," http://www.infoplease.com/ipa/A0104688.html

How Much Do You Pay Into
Medicare During a Working Life?

The authors built three models to determine how much tax our breadwinner would have paid during his lifetime, including the employer's contribution. If that 1965 breadwinner stayed in the same job for 40 years and then retired in 2005, and if his income increased at the same rate as the consumer price index, he and his employer would have paid in a total of about $16,300.[5] See Table 1 on the next page.

If our breadwinner had won a promotion every 10 years that earned him a 10 percent wage increase, when he retired in 2005, he and his employer would have paid in just a shade less than $20,000 during his lifetime.[6] See Table 2 on page 115.

We also wondered how much a middle manager who may have supervised our breadwinner would have paid in Medicare taxes during his working lifetime. Here we assumed he made $6,500 a year during 1965, $2,000 more than the breadwinner. Then we assumed that he received periodic raises at five and 10 year intervals, plus cost of living increases. If our supervisor retired in 2000, he and his employer would have paid $22,600 in Medicare taxes. If he retired at the same time as the breadwinner, the total taxes paid would have been $30,738.[7] You will find that data in Table 3 on page 116.

The Centers for Medicaid and Medicare Services indicate that it spent an average of $7,061[8] for each Medicare recipient during 2003. At that rate, our breadwinner's

---

5. "Social Security & Medicare Tax Rates," Updated December 23, 2002, U.S. Social Security Administration. Calculations for inflation are created by use of the U.S. Bureau of Labor Statistics CPI Calculator.
6. Ibid.
7. Ibid.
8. See note 2.

Year	Income	Rate x 2⁵	Ann. Total Tax	Accu. Total
1965	$4,500	.0	$0.00	$0.00
1966	$4,628	.0035	$32.40	$32.40
1967	$4,770	.005	$47.70	$80.10
1968	$4,970	.006	$59.64	$139.74
1969	$5,241	.006	$62.89	$202.63
1970	$5,541	.006	$66.49	$269.12
1971	$5,784	.006	$69.41	$338.53
1972	$5,970	.006	$71.64	$410.17
1973	$6,341	.01	$126.82	$536.99
1974	$7,040	.009	$126.72	$663.71
1975	$7,683	.009	$138.29	$802.00
1976	$8,126	.009	$146.27	$948.27
1977	$8,654	.009	$155.77	$1,104.04
1978	$9,311	.01	$186.22	$1,290.26
1979	$10,368	.0105	$217.73	$1,507.99
1980	$11,770	.0105	$247.17	$1,755.16
1981	$12,984	.013	$337.58	$2,092.74
1982	$13,779	.013	$358.25	$2,451.00
1983	$14,212	.013	$369.51	$2,820.51
1984	$14,823	.013	$385.40	$3,205.91
1985	$15,348	.0135	$414.40	$3,620.30
1986	$15,635	.0145	$453.42	$4,073.72
1987	$16,200	.0145	$469.80	$4,543.52
1988	$16,870	.0145	$489.23	$5,032.75
1989	$17,683	.0145	$512.81	$5,545.56
1990	$18,635	.0145	$540.42	$6,085.97
1991	$19,424	.0145	$563.30	$6,649.27
1992	$20,006	.0145	$580.17	$7,229.44
1993	$20,600	.0145	$597.40	$7,826.84
1994	$21,128	.0145	$612.71	$8,439.55
1995	$21,730	.0145	$630.17	$9,069.72
1996	$22,372	.0145	$648.79	$9,718.51
1997	$22,883	.0145	$663.61	$10,382.12
1998	$23,236	.0145	$673.84	$11,055.96
1999	$23,753	.0145	$688.84	$11,744.80
2000	$24,548	.0145	$711.89	$12,456.69
2001	$25,238	.0145	$731.90	$13,188.59
2002	$25,639	.0145	$743.53	$13,932.12
2003	$26,224	.0145	$760.50	$14,692.62
2004	$26,918	.0145	$780.62	$15,473.24
2005	$28,388	.0145	$823.25	$16,296.49

Table 1: Total Medicare Taxes Paid: 40-year working life; inflationary raises only

Year	Income	Rate x 2⁶	Ann. Total Tax	Accu. Total
1965	$4,500			
1966	$4,628	.0035	$32.40	$32.40
1967	$4,770	.005	$47.70	$80.10
1968	$4,970	.006	$59.64	$139.74
1969	$5,241	.006	$62.89	$202.63
1970	$5,541	.006	$66.49	$269.12
1971	$5,784	.006	$69.41	$338.53
1972	$5,970	.006	$71.64	$410.17
1973	$6,341	.01	$126.82	$536.99
1974	$7,040	.009	$126.72	$663.71
1975	$8,451	.009	$152.12	$815.53
1976	$8,939	.009	$160.89	$976.73
1977	$9,519	.009	$171.35	$1,148.08
1978	$10,242	.01	$204.84	$1,352.92
1979	$11,405	.0105	$239.50	$1,592.32
1980	$12,947	.0105	$271.89	$1,864.31
1981	$14,282	.013	$371.34	$2,235.65
1982	$15,157	.013	$394.08	$2,629.73
1983	$15,633	.013	$406.46	$3,036.19
1984	$16,305	.013	$423.94	$3,460.13
1985	$18,418	.0135	$497.28	$3,957.40
1986	$18,762	.0145	$544.10	$4,501.50
1987	$19,440	.0145	$563.76	$5,065.26
1988	$20,244	.0145	$587.08	$5,652.34
1989	$21,220	.0145	$615.37	$6,267.71
1990	$22,362	.0145	$648.50	$6,916.20
1991	$23,309	.0145	$675.96	$7,592.16
1992	$24,007	.0145	$696.21	$8,288.37
1993	$24,720	.0145	$719.88	$9,005.25
1994	$25,354	.0145	$735.25	$9,740.50
1995	$28,249	.0145	$819.22	$10,559.72
1996	$29,084	.0145	$843.42	$11,403.15
1997	$29,748	.0145	$862.69	$12,265.84
1998	$30,207	.0145	$876.00	$13,141.83
1999	$30,879	.0145	$895.49	$14,037.32
2000	$31,912	.0145	$925.46	$14,962.78
2001	$32,809	.0145	$951.47	$15,914.25
2002	$33,331	.0145	$966.59	$16,880.84
2003	$34,091	.0145	$988.64	$17,869.49
2004	$34,993	.0145	$1,014.81	$18,884.30
2005	$36,904	.0145	$1,070.23	$19,954.53

Table 2: Total Medicare Taxes Paid: 40-year Working Life; Promotions Each 10 Years, Plus Inflationary Raises Each Year

Year	Income	Rate x 2[7]	Ann. Total Tax	Accu. Total
1965	$6,500			
1966	$6,685	.0035	$46.80	$46.80
1967	$6,891	.005	$68.91	$115.71
1968	$7,180	.006	$86.16	$201.87
1969	$7,572	.006	$90.86	$292.73
1970	$8,005	.006	$96.06	$388.79
1971	$8,356	.006	$100.27	$489.06
1972	$8,624	.006	$103.49	$592.55
1973	$9,160	.01	$183.20	$775.75
1974	$10,170	.009	$183.06	$958.81
1975	$12,199	.009	$219.58	$1,178.39
1976	$12,903	.009	$232.25	$1,410.65
1977	$13,749	.009	$248.48	$1,658.13
1978	$14,794	.01	$295.88	$1,954.01
1979	$16,469	.0105	$345.85	$2,299.86
1980	$18,693	.0105	$392.55	$2,692.41
1981	$20,618	.013	$536.07	$3,228.48
1982	$21,890	.013	$569.14	$3,797.62
1983	$22,593	.013	$587.42	$4,385.04
1984	$23,565	.013	$612.69	$4,997.73
1985	$26,843	.0135	$724.76	$5,722.49
1986	$27,339	.0145	$792.83	$6,515.32
1987	$28,338	.0145	$821.80	$7,337.12
1988	$29,512	.0145	$855.85	$8,192.97
1989	$30,932	.0145	$897.03	$9,090.00
1990	$34,235	.0145	$992.82	$10,082.81
1991	$35,670	.0145	$1,034.43	$11,117.24
1992	$36,775	.0145	$1,066.48	$12,183.72
1993	$37,870	.0145	$1,098.23	$13,281.95
1994	$38,840	.0145	$1,126.36	$14,408.31
1995	$43,930	.0145	$1,273.97	$15,682.28
1996	$45,227	.0145	$1,311.58	$16,993.86
1997	$46,257	.0145	$1,341.45	$18,335.31
1998	$46,981	.0145	$1,362.45	$19,697.76
1999	$48,017	.0145	$1,392.49	$21,090.25
2000	$52,105	.0145	$1,511.05	$22,601.30
2001	$53,582	.0145	$1,553.88	$24,155.18
2002	$54,427	.0145	$1,578.38	$25,733.56
2003	$55,660	.0145	$1,614.14	$27,347.70
2004	$57,142	.0145	$1,657.12	$29,004.82
2005	$59,772	.0145	$1,733.39	**$30,738.21**

Table 3: Total Medicare Taxes Paid: 40-year Working Life; Supervisor With Four Promotions Plus Inflationary Raises

116

entire Medicare taxes would be spent in less than three years of use. Even our successful supervisor's entire taxes would be long spent after seven years upon retiring.

We know that hospital and doctor bills associated with knee replacement surgery can exceed $15,000-$20,000. Open-heart surgeries may cost more than $100,000. One major procedure will easily spend all of the Medicare tax dollars that have been paid into a person's account.

"I paid for my Medicare services while I worked," many retired people have stated, "and I should be able to spend my own money." We do not argue with the sentiment of that statement, just its total accuracy. The lifetime worker does, indeed, pay Medicare taxes and should have use of them during retirement. The total amount they pay in, however, seldom comes near the actual cost of Medicare services they receive during their retirement years.

CONGRESSIONAL ESTIMATES WERE FAR TOO LOW

From the start, Congress had grossly underestimated the real long-term cost of Medicare. "When Medicare Part A was enacted in 1965, costs were projected to rise to $9 billion by 1990, but actual costs reached $67 billion by 1990."[9] In 2003, Medicare spending reached $283 billion.[10] Medicare projections are consistently understated.

Paying Medicare's costs has increasingly become more difficult. Social Security funding helps us understand why. In 1936, when Congress passed Social Security, there were 42 taxpayers for every person who received a Social Security check. Then, "[b]ack in 1950, as the baby boom was just getting started, each retiree's benefit was divided among 16 workers. Taxes could be kept low. Today, that

9. Peter Peterson, "Remember Cost Control," *Newsweek*, July 25, 1994, as quoted in the "Cato Institute Tax and Budget Bulletin," Sept. 2003.
10. "CMS News," Centers for Medicare and Medicaid Services, Jan. 11, 2005.

number has dropped to 3.3 workers per retiree, and by 2025, it will reach – and remain at – about two workers per retiree."[11]

Does anyone really believe that, in the future, those two workers are each willingly going to give up $1,000 or more every month out of their paychecks to pay the Social Security costs of one retired baby boomer? Former Speaker of the House Newt Gingrich stated, "A transfer system, where two people are paying for a third person, is an invitation to generational warfare. Since the person who is getting the money will never think they're getting enough, and the two people who are paying will always think they're paying too much."[12]

On top of the Social Security burden lies the unfunded Medicare monster. In the next 20 years:

> Medicare spending will increase 150 percent, to $766 billion a year, whereas Social Security spending will grow 80 percent to $888 billion a year during the same time period.
>
> By 2024, Medicare costs will top those of Social Security, and by 2078, Medicare costs will double those of the retirement system.
>
> In 15 years, Medicare will require almost 25 percent of federal income tax revenue, compared to 7.5 percent today.[13]

Instead of solving the dual crises of escalating Social Security and Medicare costs, today's Congress seems intent on passing the problem to tomorrow's lawmakers.

11. Social Security Reform Center,
http://www.socialsecurityreform.org/problems/index.cfm
12. Interview with Newt Gingrich, *Limbaugh Letter*, Aug. 2005.
13. Bennett Roth, "Experts Sound Medicare Alarm: Observers say the program will be in more trouble than Social Security," *Houston Chronicle*, Feb. 6, 2005.

Both of these programs have been considered "the third rail" of politics, meaning that they are so divisive as political issues that Congress is afraid to pass real reform. Only if citizens demand change will Congress listen.

Congress, however, hears the heated hoofbeats of hundreds of thousands of Medicare enrollees who also vote in large numbers. Since 1965, they have grown accustomed to Medicare and its entitlements, and utilization of services has exploded. Congress, which created the problem in the first place, now steps in to attempt to control spending by micro-managing reimbursement rates and covered benefits.

How Medicare Tries to Control Its Spending

Medicare officials try to stretch their dollars to cover all the people aged 65 or older. They do this by setting price controls on how much Medicare will reimburse medical providers.

The prices that Medicare reimburses providers are set lower than what the insurance companies and HMOs pay for the same services. They are far lower than what uninsured persons pay.

For example, to cover all expenses, a doctor may really need to charge $96 for an office visit. Medicare sets its reimbursement rate at $64 and allows the doctor to collect another $16 from the patient. The patient might pay this directly, or his or her Medigap policy will pay the $16. If the doctor tries to collect any more than $16 from the patient, he or she can be penalized and even barred from seeing Medicare patients.

If the doctor needs $96 per patient to cover all the clinic's expenses, and can only collect $80, a shortage of $16 must be paid by someone. The doctor, then, must collect

$112 from people younger than age 65, either through their insurance, or directly from people who have high deductible insurance policies or are uninsured. The clinic negotiates reimbursement rates with insurance companies that average about 40 percent above the Medicare rate, but the clinic often sets the "retail price" of its service higher than the insurance rate. So the price charged to uninsured persons might be $128, or even higher.

The reason, then, that health insurance premiums are able to drop by 70 percent or more for a Medicare patient is because all working people and their employers pay taxes on earned income to fund Medicare. They help pay the Medicare recipient's premium cost. Medicare then pays the least amount possible to health care providers and makes it unlawful for providers to collect anything above that set amount.

You might suggest that the government should just set the cost of health care for everyone at the Medicare rate, that they should control prices the same way as many foreign governments do. If Congress did this, and such a law somehow passed the scrutiny of the U.S. Supreme Court, then every American would receive $80 health care instead of $112 health care. Clinics would have to find a way to slash their expenses by reducing the quality of health care, while creating shortages and long waiting lines. Americans are fussy about the quality of health care and would never tolerate discount doctoring.

As Medicare is structured today, Americans older than 64 and those who are approaching that age can look forward to reduced out-of-pocket health care insurance costs. Younger workers, however, have grave concerns as they pay almost all of the Medicare taxes; and because of cost shifting, pay more for their own health care services.

MEDICARE SPENDING GREW 16 PERCENT A YEAR
FOR 10 YEARS FOLLOWING THE CREATION OF HMOS

As spending began to spiral out of control after Medicare became effective, Congress wanted seniors to enroll in HMOs and offered them a choice. They could stay in the fee-for-service plans to which they had become accustomed, or move to HMOs. The idea of breaking a life-long relationship with a family doctor or losing the ability to choose which specialists to see, did not appeal to many seniors at first. HMOs, on the other hand, offered almost unlimited preventive care, plus a prescription drug benefit. This attracted millions of enrollees.

The premium charged for an increased number of benefits under an HMO plan was the same or even lower than a fee-for-service policy. The enrollee had to assign their Medicare benefits to the HMO.

The government's strategy to use the gatekeeper doctor to control cost, however, backfired. HMO-enrollees paid little to nothing to see the doctor. From infrequent doctor visits prior to the creation of Medicare, when patients paid for each visit out of their own pocket, HMO care reduced or removed all personal financial restraint, and seniors took advantage of it like anyone else would do. At the extreme, some seniors even found that going to the doctor reduced their loneliness. Health spending exploded. Medicare spending grew 15.8 percent a year for the 10 years following the creation of HMOs.[14]

Traditional insurance companies that offered fee-for-service policies were forced to offer more benefits to compete with HMOs. Yet, they also had to hold their premiums steady. Some insurance companies quit selling to seniors. After a time, many seniors came to resent being controlled

---

14. See note 2.

by the gatekeeper doctor. Many complained that the gate-keepers were preventing them from much-needed care, just to hold down spending. They wanted the freedom to choose their own specialists, and participate with their doctor in the design of treatment plans. They chose to go back to fee-for-service plans, even though they had to give up some preventive care, and pay a higher monthly premium.

As pharmaceutical companies continued to introduce expensive new "miracle" drugs, political pressure mounted to provide relief to cash-strapped seniors to help pay their prescription drug costs. The media and senior advocacy groups began to report about seniors who had to choose between eating dog food, or purchasing life-supporting drugs. Bipartisan political support gelled in 2003 to add a prescription drug benefit to Medicare – Part D.

MEDICARE PART D:
THE 2003 MEDICARE MODERNIZATION ACT – PRESCRIPTION DRUG COVERAGE, AN UNTOLD TRUTH

Political considerations drove the passage of the 2003 Medicare Modernization Act, which featured prescription drug coverage for seniors. In 2004, Republican President George W. Bush faced a difficult reelection challenge, as did every member of the U.S. House of Representatives, and one-third of the senators. Democrats have long been seen as the party that cares for senior citizens, and seniors' groups had worked for a long time to win a prescription drug benefit for Medicare enrollees. Acting shrewdly, President Bush and the Republicans in Congress made sure that the new drug benefit passed before the 2004 election cycle, thus taking it off the table as a political debate. Sen. John Kerry, the Democratic candidate for president in 2004, faced the daunting task of convincing seniors that Pres. Bush had failed them, even though the president had been aligned clearly with this politically popular reform.

When the American Association of Retired Persons (AARP) signed on to the 2003 legislation, it assured its passage. Those voices that opposed the law and worried about its real costs were muffled.

The <u>unspoken truth</u> is that the 2003 prescription drug plan is a near duplicate of H.R. 3600, the 1994 Health Care bill, often called HillaryCare.[15] This is the bill that resulted from Mrs. Clinton's health care study group, and that Americans soundly rejected during the 1994 election. Having failed to convince the U.S. voters to turn over all of health care to public control, the politicians have adopted a strategy of incrementalism.

Incrementalism is a strategy whereby small parts of unpopular ideas are slowly adopted, in such a way that very few people will realize what is being done to them. This strategy is demonstrated by the story of how to boil a live frog. You place the frog into a pot of cool water, and slowly turn up the heat. The frog never notices that the heat is increasing, until it is too late, and the pot has boiled away his life. That is incrementalism.

From its inception, nearly all sides of the argument admitted that the 2003 law was far from perfect, and left everyone hoping for future incremental law changes. As many advocates for U.S. seniors acknowledge privately, if the bill had not passed in 2003, it may have never passed. They knew that once the cost of covering Baby Boomers had been factored in, the program costs would explode. By passing it in 2003, they could avoid a public debate about the program's true long-term costs.

Free market advocates were able to win a few conces-

---

15. H.R. 3600, 103rd Congress, line 3 & following, 351.

sions. Primarily this meant allowing multiple health insurance companies to offer Part D drug coverage. Competitive pressures between insurance companies should serve to hold down costs.

To fully understand Part D benefits, you can call a local health insurance agent, or go to websites sponsored by insurance companies. Our website also provides links. Go to www.yourhealthmattersbook.com.

WHO REALLY NEEDED PART D AND WHO REALLY BENEFITS?

Myth: Low-income Americans needed Part D to help them purchase drugs.

Truth: Low-income Americans already had government programs to help them purchase drugs under state Medicaid programs.[16]

Why did Congress create this plan? For whom was it trying to deliver this new benefit?

Low-income seniors on Medicare were not falling through the cracks. They were already able to get the prescriptions they needed under state Medicaid programs at very low, or even no cost (Medicaid is covered in the next chapter).

So if low-income Americans didn't need Part D coverage, who then would benefit from this new entitlement program? The general population believed that countless seniors were unable to purchase life-saving drugs. Medicare Part D, however, is actually designed to provide reimbursements to middle- and upper-income people. It is done without any income or asset test – every Medicare enrollee is eligible. Congress, the president, the media, and seniors' advocacy groups had made it seem like a crisis for all sen-

16. "Medicaid At-a-Glance, 2003," A Medicaid Information Source, Centers for Medicare and Medicaid Services, 10.

iors, and claimed it was unfair to deny prescription drugs to them. Is it fair, however, that lower income workers should help buy drugs for wealthy retired persons?

Bill Gates, the richest man in the world, will qualify for Medicare at age 65, despite the fact that his personal net worth exceeds that of some foreign governments. If he needs prescription drugs and chooses to exercise his right to enroll in Medicare Part D, why should Microsoft's janitors be forced to pay Medicare taxes to support Bill Gates' benefit?

Part D could, however, provide Americans who take drugs each day a great savings. For those with extremely high drug costs, the program will save them thousands of dollars a year. About 75 percent of the Medicare Part D cost must be subsidized by taxes on working people; those who participate in Part D will pay about 25 percent of the actual cost of the insurance.[17]

The Medicare Part D prescription drug program will face numerous changes during the next several decades. It is a sure bet that it will cost far in excess of $700 billion in the next 10 years, as the politicians asserted.

Once again, government has distorted market forces by subsidizing health care costs, and by insulating consumers from the true cost of their prescriptions. This will result in increased use of pharmaceuticals, their price will go up, and all of this will force overall health care spending even higher. There are free market alternatives, which we discuss in chapter 10.

A FEW PARTING THOUGHTS

Medicare insurance has delivered high-quality, affordable, and needed health care to millions of Americans.

17. Peter, Ashkenaz, Deputy Director, CMS Media, Centers for Medicare and Medicaid, via email, Feb. 13, 2006.

Those who think ahead to retirement are counting on it to provide the bulk of their health care needs. It is obviously impossible to know what would have happened if Medicare had never been created, and if the United States would have allowed the free market to find solutions for senior health care issues.

There are serious short- and long-term financing problems with Medicare, and the financial pain is felt by the workers who pay its costs. Even before the Part D drug plan was added in 2003, Congress knew that the United States faced a huge unfunded Medicare deficit. "The latest Medicare trustees' report shows the long-term cost of Medicare's unfunded promises jumped roughly $2 trillion in just one year and the debt for the drug benefit alone jumped from $8.1 trillion to $8.7 trillion."[18]

What has happened with Medicare is common to the government-gatekeeper systems favored by many foreign nations (see chapter 14). They, too, face runaway spending for their aging populations, knowing that high usage always follows the perception that health care is free.

Medicare started out 40 years ago to provide health insurance to about three percent of the population, those seniors who did not own health insurance. Since then, it has grown to be a comprehensive entitlement program, serving 41 million people, with the only qualifying factor that the enrollee must be age 65.

Medicare has had the profound effect of changing the social attitude of Americans from one of self-reliance to one of government dependence.

---

18. Robert E. Moffit, Ph.D. and Andrew Grossman, "Defusing the Medicare Time Bomb," The Heritage Foundation, May 26, 2005.

CHAPTER 9
MEDICAID
HEALTH CARE FOR LOW- AND MIDDLE- INCOME AMERICANS

When Medicaid started in 1965, good-hearted Americans wanted it to help a limited number of low-income people younger than 65 pay for their basic health care needs.

Medicaid entitled people with few financial assets to access a basic set of necessary health care services. From its original limited mission, however, it has exploded into an extended maze of overlapping programs that deliver health care services to more than 36.5 million people.

Federal and state governments spent $267 billion[1] for Medicaid programs during 2003. Added to that, various government units spent another $216 billion on health care programs,[2] for a total of $483 billion on non-Medicare services.

The total non-Medicare spending of $483 billion startled the authors. We compared it to total health care spending funded by the private sector, at $913 billion.[3] We wanted to calculate the cost of health care per person spent by the private sector versus government programs, but the

---

1. "Health Care Spending in the United States Slows for the First Time in Seven Years," *CMS News,* Centers for Medicare and Medicaid Services, Jan. 11, 2005.
2. Ibid.
3. Ibid.

Centers for Medicare and Medicaid refuse to disclose it. They say in a footnote, "Calculation of per capita estimates is inappropriate."[4] We see nothing inappropriate about our government telling us how much of our tax dollars are spent per person to provide free or subsidized health care.

The authors wanted to understand why government health care programs appear to cost so much more than non-government funded programs. Did it have something to do with the health of the population it served? Could the population have been mostly severely disabled persons? We knew that those with chronic illnesses consume a large amount of health care, but certainly, the tens of millions who receive health care paid for by the government cannot all be chronically severely ill.

We went to government sources to find the answers. There we encountered a maze of programs, regulations, requirements, data sources, and thousands of pages of information. Each page referred us to a number of other pages, which referred us to yet another set of sources, in an endless and futile search for answers. Each one of these sources, we knew, required the work of a number of government employees. We could only conclude that one of the major reasons government-provided health care is so expensive is the administrative costs required to operate the bureaucracy.

We doubt that anyone really understands it all, and that is why it seems out of control. We did find, however, that Medicaid provides an extended health benefit set even to many middle-income families. This varies state by state.

QUALIFYING INCOME LEVELS

States set their own income and asset guidelines for

4. "Table 4: Personal Health Care Expenditures Aggregate and Per Capita Amounts and Distribution, by Source of Funds: Selected Calendar Years 1980-2003," Centers for Medicare and Medicaid Services, U.S. Government. footnote

those who qualify for Medicaid. Some states pay benefits to people who have incomes up to 150 percent of the federal poverty threshold. Other states provide Medicaid to middle-income persons earning as much as 275 or even 280 percent of the federal poverty threshold (see Table 1 on the next page).

In a single-parent family with three children younger than 18, the poverty threshold for 2005 is $19,350. This family could receive Medicaid health care coverage if the family income was as high as $53,213 in some states. There may be additional government programs to help pay other health care costs not covered by Medicaid. As well, these families are often eligible for other government programs, such as food stamps, rent subsidies, educational programs, and job training. The definition of needy has obviously changed radically since Medicaid's inception. So has the definition of basic health care benefits.

COVERED BENEFITS

These are the services the federal government requires each state to offer under Medicaid to people who qualify because of their lack of income:[5]

- hospital, physician, medical, and surgical dental services;
- nursing facility or home health care services for individuals aged 21 or older;
- family planning services and supplies (in some states, this means paying for abortions and contraceptives);

---

5. "Medicaid At-a Glance, 2005; A Medicaid Information Source," Centers for Medicare and Medicaid Services, 4-5.
6. Ibid., 6.

Family Members	Poverty Threshold	150% Above Threshold	175% Above Threshold	200% Above Threshold	250% Above Threshold	275% Above Threshold
1	$9,570	$14,355	$16,748	$19,140	$23,925	$26,318
2	$12,830	$19,245	$22,453	$25,660	$32,075	$35,283
3	$16,090	$24,135	$28,158	$32,180	$40,225	$44,248
4	$19,350	$29,025	$33,863	$38,700	$48,375	$53,213
5	$22,610	$33,915	$39,568	$45,220	$56,525	$62,178
6	$25,870	$38,805	$45,273	$51,740	$64,675	$71,143
7	$29,130	$43,695	$50,978	$58,260	$72,825	$80,108
8	$32,390	$48,585	$56,683	$64,780	$80,975	$89,073

Table 1: Family Size, Poverty Thresholds and State Income Qualification Levels[6]

- some rural health clinic and ambulatory services;
- laboratory and x-ray services;
- pediatric and family nurse practitioner services;
- some federally-qualified health center services and any other ambulatory services offered by a federally-qualified health center;
- some nurse-midwife services; and
- early and periodic screening, diagnosis, and treatment services for individuals under age 21.

Some states also choose to cover certain categories of people under Medicaid based on types of health problems. In these cases, the federal government requires that the state plan, as a minimum, cover the following services:

- prenatal care and delivery services for pregnant women;
- ambulatory services to individuals under age 18 and individuals entitled to institutional services;
- home health services to individuals entitled to nursing facility services; and
- some services for those labeled mentally retarded.

Some states also offer optional services, the most common of which are:

- clinic services;
- nursing facility services for those under age 21;

- intermediate care facility/mentally retarded services;
- optometrist services and eyeglasses;
- prescribed drugs (every state offers this);
- TB-related services for TB-infected persons;
- prosthetic devices; and
- dental services.

From what began as a limited set of health-sustaining benefits, in a great majority of the states Medicaid now offers comprehensive health care benefits. In some states, the benefits are more generous than what is available to those people who pay for their own health insurance or receive it through their employers.

The Medicaid patient feels entitled to consume health care without concern for cost. And why not? Taxpayers pay the bills, not the Medicaid patient. This might also be a reason for the high cost per person on Medicaid.

Each state has customized their health care programs for low-income persons. You can check out your own state by going to www.yourhealthmattersbook.com and linking to the Centers for Medicare and Medicaid. There you can select your state. You may also want to compare your state to others.

States pay a portion of the Medicaid health care costs, and the federal government pays the balance. The amount each state pays ranges from 50 percent to just 23% (in Mississippi).[7] State Medicaid programs have become the second largest budget item for most states, and may become the largest, even greater than that of children's education.

---

7. See note 5, 7.

SOME STATES EVEN TRY TO COMPETE

Many state governments have come to believe that only they can make sure that everyone has access to health insurance.

Some states have even felt the need to go into the health insurance business. They claim that their insurance plan offers low premium cost, and high quality comprehensive insurance. Minnesota, for instance, has offered its MinnesotaCare program since 1993. Its costs are paid by a two percent "sick tax" assessed on all health care charges. MinnesotaCare offers reduced and subsidized premiums based on income and number of dependents. The insurance works quite well until someone gets seriously ill or injured. What the MinnesotaCare application form fails to disclose is its $10,000 calendar year limit on payments to hospitals, and $5,000 for doctor charges, for adult enrollees. One hospital trip of just a day or two would easily exceed that limit, and send the insured person into bankruptcy.

What is most curious about MinnesotaCare's undisclosed spending limit is that most persons can purchase a $1,500 deductible Blue Cross policy for substantially less, and enjoy the security of a $3 million lifetime benefit. For example, an adult earning $25,600 pays an annual premium of $2,520 for MinnesotaCare coverage.[8] In the private insurance market, a 19-year-old male could purchase a Blue Cross policy for $1,218, a 34-year-old for $1,350, a 44-year-old for $1,572, and a 49-year-old, for $1,962.[9] Purchasing the Blue Cross policy would save premium dollars and add far more security and protection. Yet more than 33,700[10] adults in Minnesota have opted for MinnesotaCare, likely unaware that they could purchase far better

---

8. MinnesotaCare Premium Table, July 2005 - June 2006, 4.
9. Blue Cross, Blue Shield, Minnesota Rate Sheet, 2005.
10. Warren Wolfe, "For Some A Painful Cut," *Minneapolis Star-Tribune,* Jan. 31, 2005.

insurance for less money in the private market.

A $1 million lifetime benefit was mandated by Minnesota state law[11] as the minimum amount to be a qualified health plan.[12] That law was written by the same legislature that put the $10,000 cap on MinnesotaCare. Perhaps they knew that the state insurance product, without its severe limits, could not compete with private health insurance.

Meanwhile, those who advocate a government takeover of health care, publicly chastise providers for aggressively seeking reimbursements from persons who do not pay their health care bills, many of whom could be MinnesotaCare enrollees.

SPECIAL KIDS CARE

Congress also created the State Children's Health Insurance Program – SCHIP – as a state-based program. It hoped to solve the problem of leaving American children uninsured.

Most poor children are covered under Medicaid, if their parents are covered. Yet there are children whose parents earn too much to be covered under Medicaid, but do not buy health insurance for their children. Children who live in families with incomes below 200 percent of the federal poverty threshold might be able to be covered under SCHIP.

Many states receive Medicaid and SCHIP funds, and then roll them into their own state-based health care plans (like MinnesotaCare).[13]

Community health centers were also part of the 1960s federal health care initiatives. CHCs provide billions of

---

11. MN Statutes, 62E04, 62E06.
12. A qualified plan is one in which an employer is able to receive a state income tax deduction on the health insurance premium it pays on behalf of its employees.
13. See note 5, 3.

dollars a year of subsidized health care to low-income and uninsured people. (See chapter 13 that deals with the uninsured question.)

Another program that states run that is paid for partly by federal taxes is called the Maternal and Child Health (MCH) Benefit. The federal government spent nearly $1 billion on this program in 2003. Its purpose is to improve the health of women, children, youth, and families. MCH, like Medicaid, is a state and federal partnership.

TIME TO CHANGE

Governments spent more than $766 billion[14] for health care in 2003. That amounts to 46 percent of all health care spending. As of the end of 2003, there were 130 million working Americans[15] and another 10.3 million self-employed people.[16] These 140.3 million people pay the bulk of Medicare and income taxes. The cost of these programs average $5,460 per working person each year.[17] A portion of these payments are, of course, recovered through Medicare and Medigap premiums, co-payments and co-insurance. Even if these payments covered 50 percent of the cost, the working person and his or her employer would still be responsible for $2,800 a year in various taxes to subsidize health care for other people. Working families and their employers are already paying thousands of dollars a year in health insurance premium, and also carry the tax burden of those who receive government health care benefits.

The simple fact is that 77 million Americans use Medicare and Medicaid programs and the costs are sky-

---

14. See note 1.
15. http://www.bls.gov/oes/current/oes_00A1.htm
16. http://www.bls.gov/eps/wlf-table36-2005.pdf
17. $766 billion divided by 140.3 million working people.

rocketing. On the one hand, some health care reformers believe that more people should be covered under these federal programs – such as lowering the Medicare age to 55. Others believe that the only way to solve the problem is to put the federal government in charge of everyone's health care. Still others believe that these two federal programs threaten the United States' economic stability and security.

For certain, before governments expend any more effort trying to reform private health care and private health insurance, the authors believe it needs to clean up its own programs. There is no reason for U.S. residents to accept the government's leadership when the government has not demonstrated its ability to deliver care to those who need it at a reasonable cost.

We want our elected officials to account for their use of tax dollars spent to provide free or subsidized health care. Of that $766 billion, how much was actually paid to the doctors, hospitals, drug companies, and other health care providers who cared for Medicare, Medicaid and other types of patients? Knowing the amount paid to the providers would reveal the hidden cost of government administration. Then we would know how much actually ends up paying for health care, and better understand why, or if, health care spending for government-subsidized care is far more than that provided by private sources.

CHAPTER 10
WONDER DRUGS:
IT'S A WONDER THAT
WE CAN AFFORD THEM

Question: Why do prescription drugs cost so much? Aren't there any alternatives to expensive drugs that people can afford? Doesn't the high price of drugs play a major role in the explosion of U.S. health care spending? Can't we just import drugs from Canada or elsewhere and save big money?

"U.S. prescription drug sales grew 8.3 percent to $235.4 billion in 2004, compared with $217.3 billion in sales the previous year."[1] This equals about 14 percent of our total spending on U.S. health care.

The cost of prescription drugs is increasing at a more rapid pace than any other segment of the health care market. In the years leading up to 2004, total spending on prescription drugs had risen more than 10 percent for several straight years.

Worldwide, prescription drug sales exceeded $550 bil-

---

1. "IMS Reports 8.3 Percent Dollar Growth in 2004 U.S. Prescription Sales," Feb. 14, 2005. http://www.imshealth.com/ims/portal/front/articles/ O,27777,6599_40183881_74240066,00.html

lion during 2004. Every foreign health care system struggles to pay its country's prescription drug bills (see chapter 14).

Truly, prescription drugs are big business. As much as they relieve pain and suffering while extending life, for those who pay the health care bill, they create pain in the pocketbook.

SO LET'S LOOK NORTH –
EVERYONE KNOWS CANADIANS HAVE IT BETTER;
OR DO THEY?

Myth: Canadians pay less for name brand drugs because they have a single-payer health care system, run by the government.

Unspoken Secret: Health Canada and its provincial government drug plans require a high out-of-pocket cost before insurance pays for the bulk of prescriptions.

Health Canada, the national health plan of Canada, does not cover prescription drugs for most of its citizens, except for some specific groups of persons (Intuit Indians, low-income people, etc.). Each province administers its own drug plan under minimum guidelines set by Health Canada.

From what all of us have been told by U.S. media, Canada appears to have been successful in making drugs more affordable for their citizens than what the United States has been able to do. As the media present the case, Americans are charged unfair high prices, and as a result, tens of thousands of U.S. residents now order their drugs from Canadian pharmacies.

In Canada, name brand drugs sell for less because individuals have to pay for their own drugs, or sign up for a provincial prescription drug plan. Canadian prescription drug coverage varies from province to province, and is far different from that offered in the United States.

The Fair PharmaCare coverage in British Columbia is representative of the plans in the other provinces. For families, the plan pays nothing until the family has spent $1,000, the plan's deductible. After paying the $1,000 deductible, the Canadian still must pay the first 30 percent of the cost of each prescription until they spend four percent of their total family income.

A Canadian family that earns $32,000 could pay as much as $2,280 out-of-pocket ($1,000 deductible plus four percent of $32,000) before insurance pays the balance of their drug costs. No U.S. non-Medicare insurance plan has a $1,000 deductible to meet, and co-pays are usually $10 or $25; seldom more.

Compare the out-of-pocket costs of Lipitor. Americans pay a maximum of $10-$25 a month of the $100 a month cost. A Canadian will pay the $1,000 deductible (10 months worth); during the rest of the year, the Canadian will pay $30 a month for the drug. The American pays between $120 and $300 for a year's supply, while the Canadian pays as much as $1,060.

Since Canadians must pay so much of their own drug costs, even if they own prescription drug insurance, the drug companies must meet the price that people are willing or able to pay. Drug companies know how much Canadian citizens are willing to spend on name brand drugs. Canadians spend less because they pay more of the costs directly. Therefore, drug companies must agree to an affordable price with Health Canada.

Unspoken Secret: Canadians know what their drugs cost, and Americans do not, because Canadians pay so much of the upfront cost of their drugs.

Drug	Canada[2]	United States[3]	%-less cost for Canadian drug
Lipitor 20 mg, 50 capsules	$212.34	$305.19	30 percent less
Prosac[4] 10 mg capsules	$189.73	$365.87	48 percent less
Nexium[5] 20 mg	$87.77	$139.99	37 percent less
Coumadin 3 mg, 100 capsules	$52.60	$81.99	36 percent less

Table 1: Price Comparison of Selective Drugs; U.S. and Canada
Prosac cannot be sold across the border. It is shown only as an example of a popular drug for comparative pricing purposes.

All prices are in U.S. dollars.

Canadian prices for name brand drugs can be significantly less than what Americans pay for the same product. Table 1 gives an example.

If the U.S. government and insurance companies had adopted the Canadian strategy of not subsidizing the majority of prescription drug costs, American drug prices would fall. Instead, the U.S. government has instituted a costly massive drug subsidy program – Medicare Part D – that will further insulate U.S. residents from the true cost of their drugs.

Health Canada, paradoxically, has interfered with generic drug pricing. This has forced their citizens to pay far more for generics than they should.

ACTUALLY, CANADIANS MAY PAY MUCH MORE

Unspoken Secret: Canadians pay two to three times as much for generic drugs and over-the-counter medicines as Americans do.

---

2. http://www.CanadaDrugs.com, June 23, 2005
3. http://www.walgreens.com, June 23, 2005
4. CanadaDrugs.com sells 100 capsules while Walgreens sells 90 capsules. Price has been adjusted to reflect this difference.
5. CanadaDrugs.com sells 28 tablets while Walgreens sells 30 tablets. Price has been adjusted to reflect this difference.

A comprehensive study showed that for the 27 most commonly used generic drugs, "Canadian generic prices were on average more than double the prices charged in the U.S."[6] If Canadians could buy generic drugs as cheaply as Americans do, they would have saved C$400 million during 2001. To provide perspective, a Canadian savings of C$400 million is the same as the U.S. saving $2.9 billion.

"Considering half of all drugs sold in the United States are generic, it is surprising how little attention has been paid to them in the reimportation debate."[7]

In the U.S., generics cost about 74 percent less than name brand drugs, but in Canada, they are only 38 percent less. Generics offer a great savings for Americans, but a greater cost for Canadians.

The U.S. Food and Drug Administration (FDA) conducted an experiment during 2004 concerning generic drug prices. Federal officials had seized a large number of Canadian drug shipments that came through the Bahamas. Discounting charges for freight, the FDA compared the Canadian prices with what Americans would have paid for the same drugs at a corner drug store. Those Americans who had ordered their generics from Canada paid 67 percent more than if they had bought the same drugs here.[8]

Canada prohibits the free market from saving its citizens money on generics by limiting competition, and price fixing. "...[T]wo companies (Apotex and Novopharm) account for more than half of the total Canadian generic market."[9] In the U.S., once a drug has lost its patent protection, dozens of generic drug manufacturers will make it available, driving down the price.

---

6. "Generic Drug Prices, a Canada-US Comparison," Palmer D'Angelo Consulting Inc., Aug. 2002.
7. John Goodman, "Free trade tack for drug imports," *The Washington Times*, Jan. 31, 2005
8. U.S./Canadian Price Comparisons, Oct. 2004,
http://www.fda.gov/oc/opacom/hottopics/importdrugs/CanadaRX.html
9. See note 7.

Canadian provinces have fixed generic drug prices in a way that keeps them artificially high. "The Ontario Drug Benefit Plan has established rules that require the first generic entrant to be priced at 70% of the brand price and subsequent entrants at 63% of the brand."[10] (It is hard to understand why Health Canada would want to keep generic drug prices artificially high. Perhaps they agree to set these prices high as a negotiating tool, used to win lower prices for name brand drugs. Still, it robs Canadians of the chance to save hundreds of dollars on less expensive generics in favor of the more expensive name brand drugs.)

The low-cost of generic drugs in the United States plays a sizable role in holding down overall health care spending. "Generic products account for less than 10 percent of total sales for the U.S. prescription drug market but 51 percent of the total prescriptions filled."[11] That is, more than half of all drugs consumed by Americans are generic, but their cost is only 10 percent of the total that we spend on drugs. They sell at an average cost of 74 percent less than name brand drugs. America's freer markets in generics, without government price fixing, keeps our generic prices down.

Canada has taken advantage of the free market by not paying the total cost of name brand prescription drugs, and this has the result of holding their cost down. Yet, at the same time, they have interfered with the generic drug market by limiting competition and price-fixing. In the U.S. we reverse this. U.S. health care payers offer a prescription drug entitlement that shields people from the actual cost of the drugs, but allows the free market to offer very affordable, even inexpensive, generic drugs.

---

10. See note 6.
11. Christine Provost Peters, "Fundamentals of the Prescription Drug Market," NHPF Background Paper, Aug. 24, 2004.

Once again, we see how government intervention in the free market system causes spiraling health care costs. Americans also pay much less than Canadians for over-the-counter drugs and medicines.

SAVING HUGE DOLLARS ON DRUGS

Unspoken Secret: The free market can drive the cost of drugs down dramatically – even as 98 percent or more.

Wonder drugs, such as Allegra, Flonase, and Claritin have brought incredible relief to allergy sufferers. When they first came out, the retail price of these drugs ranged from $75-200 a month. Most insurance plans covered at least one of these drugs. Insured persons only paid the co-payment of $10-$25 each month. People without drug coverage either paid the retail price or went without.

Then in 2002, the FDA approved Claritin for sale over the counter (OTC). OTC drugs are purchased without a prescription, and, most importantly, OTC drugs are not covered by insurance. This affected hundreds of thousands of insured persons who used Claritin and the other drugs. Instead of paying their $10-$25 co-payment, they now realized that the retail price was as much as $75. Claritin knew that their new OTC price would have to come close to what people had gotten used to paying. Not surprisingly, the price of OTC Claritin became $25 to $30 a month.

When Claritin's patent protection expired, generic competitors came in to gain a share of the market. The results were astonishing. The price eventually dropped to about $1.20 a month. Currently consumers can buy an entire year's supply of OTC Loradatine, the generic version of Claritin, for as little as $14 *a year* at Costco.[12] This is greater than 98 percent less than the original price of

---

12. Priced by telephone call on Dec. 3, 2005, Costco, Eden Prairie, MN.

name brand Claritin that insurance companies and the government were paying for just five years ago.

This Claritin experience shows us how free markets can drive costs down, while maintaining quality. It demonstrates the proper role that government plays in protecting your health, as they made sure that OTC Claritin was both effective and safe without a doctor's prescription. Of course, before we could get to this point, Claritin had to spend hundreds of millions of dollars to develop their product, and their patent protected them long enough to recover their investment and earn a profit, and give them incentive to develop another new, breakthrough wonder drug for tomorrow.

Still, why do prescription drugs have to cost so much?

BLAME BIG PHARMA?

The drug companies – Big Pharma – are often labeled villains. They catch blame for the spike in drug costs and are sued if their drug hurts someone.

We have come to believe that the drug companies charge too much, and some want the U.S. government to force down prices. Many Americans believe that Big Pharma uses its money to pressure politicians to leave them alone, or give them special protection.

We see drug companies as so profit-driven that they ignore public safety about deadly failures of their drugs, like Vioxx. The fact is that when someone sues and collects, the consumer, once again is isolated from the true costs. Those costs, however, must be added to the cost of health care.

In chapter 6, Defensive Doctoring, we referred to the Robert Ernst case. A Texas jury had awarded his widow $253 million in a settlement with Merck, the manufacturer of Vioxx. Merck had sold Vioxx as an effective pain killer for those suffering with debilitating, chronic pain.

During September 2004, the Merck Company voluntarily pulled Vioxx off the market. Merck had learned that Vioxx might contribute to strokes, heart attacks, and death. Once the Vioxx story broke, follow-up news stories, editorials, and letters to the editor accused Merck officials of being capitalists more interested in profits than in really helping anyone. Their stock immediately dropped 27 percent in value. Trial lawyers set up websites and ran advertisements to recruit people to sue Merck. Merck now faces more than 5,000 lawsuits, and the company will be tied up in court for years.

Merck's Vioxx problem became public with the release of a report of a three-year study of 1,300 people who took the drug. The study found 15 Vioxx users (1.2 percent) who suffered either a heart attack, stroke, or died. Since the patient had been taking Vioxx at the time of their distress, some investigators believed that the drug played a role in those events. Not willing to take any more risks, Merck pulled the drug off the market.

Medical device manufacturers face similar legal liability challenges as drug companies do. During June 2005, and for months afterward, stories of a handful of deaths related to the malfunction of a defibrillator manufactured by the Guidant Corporation sent its sales and stock plummeting. A defibrillator, a device implanted in the chest, is designed to shock the heart if it quits beating. The failure rate of Guidant defibrillators stood at less than .2 (two-tenths) percent of the total sold. When it comes to personal safety, the public has zero tolerance for errors.

A child who would have otherwise died without a pacemaker suddenly discovers the one inside him might stop working. A 90-year old Grandma whose pacemaker has worked properly for several years now worries that it will short-circuit – and complications from replacement surgery might cause her death.

One device or drug failure resulting in death creates a scandal that costs companies like Guidant and Merck hundreds of millions of dollars in losses.

When you read stories about Vioxx or the Guidant defibrillator, you may become angry with Big Drug companies, and find fault with everything about them. Here is the rest of the story.

ARE DRUGS ANY GOOD?

"For millions of Americans, prescription drugs save lives, ease suffering, reduce disability, and restore vitality. Vaccines have virtually eliminated the threat of horrible diseases, such as polio, diphtheria, and whooping cough, that once made childhood a more precarious time of life. Protease inhibitors can commute the death sentence that HIV infection once conferred; antipsychotic medications allow many mentally ill persons to live full, productive lives in their communities; and beta blockers can help prevent repeated heart attacks."[13]

No wonder we Americans spend so much money on drugs and medical devices. They have improved the lives of tens of millions of people and saved the lives of hundreds of thousands of others. They eliminate or postpone dangerous and expensive surgical procedures, and can hold down costs associated with other invasive treatments.

Not only have prescription drugs performed well for so many, the future holds more exciting breakthroughs. "Advances in science such as gene therapy, cell regeneration, therapeutic cloning, and the completion of the human

---

13. See note 11.

genome sequencing provide hope for the prevention and treatment of disease in the future."[14] However, long before these scientific advances reach the public as drugs or devices, their manufacturers will have spent hundreds of millions of dollars creating them. Once on the market, the companies hope that doctors will prescribe them, and that they can turn a reasonable profit before their patent protection runs out.

RESEARCH AND DEVELOPMENT

To create new drugs requires an immense investment of money into research and development (R&D). For every 10 new products that "innovator" drug companies try to develop, only three will sell well enough to pay all the R&D costs. "The revenues from these [few successful] products must pay not only for the investment costs of the successful products but for the ones that fail as well."[15]

Just in 2002, the drug companies spent a combined $32 billion on R&D, about 16 percent of their total sales. It takes 12-15 years to take a new drug from an idea all the way to the market, and it is very expensive. "Cutting Edge..., a private sector industry monitor, estimated the cost as $900 million."[16]

Though many new drugs start from scratch, others are adapted from drugs that are already on the market. These types of drugs have an average cost of $108 million.[17]

"The majority of new drug applications approved by the FDA each year are for drugs that are modified versions of existing approved drugs..."[18] These are newer versions

---

14. Ibid.
15. Ibid.
16. Joan Buckley and Seamus OL Tuama, "International pricing and distribution of therapeutic pharmaceuticals: an ethical minefield," *Business Ethics, A European Review, Vol. 14, No. 5,* April 2005, 131.
17. Ibid.
18. See note 11.

of an older drug, often one that is about to lose its patent protection. By making minor changes in the formulation, or by developing different dosages or ways to deliver the drug (liquid versus pill form, pill form versus injection, etc.), a manufacturer, in a sense, invents a "new product" and might win additional patent protection. This reduces the cost of development for that new and improved, or just different, version.

The $900 million investment does not include tax breaks, taxpayer-funded research, and other considerations that should be factored into the true development costs. Still, when drug companies develop a true, innovator, "blockbuster" drug, the costs run to hundreds of millions of dollars, without any assurance that they will ever sell a single pill.

FDA approval of innovator drugs has slowed in recent years. In 2003, the FDA approved only 21, compared with 35 in 1999. In some ways, this is because many of the easier drugs to develop have already been completed. The drug companies now must focus on more exotic and expensive drugs, and on new types of treatment.

GOVERNMENT'S ROLE

The United States Constitution gives the federal government the responsibility to protect patents and copyrights. As such, Congress writes laws that give drug companies and medical device manufacturers protection for their innovations. Congress realizes that Americans gain from the development of new drugs and medical devices, and patent protection helps to make it possible for capitalists to risk their money.

Federal law provides 20 years of U.S. patent protection for new drugs, and the World Trade Organization members have pledged to respect these patents. In theory, this means that once a patent is secured, the drug company has the exclusive right to manufacture and market that drug all across the world. When the patent expires, the generic drug companies can make their inexpensive versions. Other name brand companies often try to make copycat drugs that sell for less than the original name brand price because those companies are able to spend less on R&D.

Patent protection is required to ensure that drug companies have a chance to recover their R&D costs and to provide investors with a return on investment. Without that protection, new drugs would not be created by private industry.

In reality, though, most companies do not enjoy 20 years of patent protection. They often receive their patents early on in the development process, and by the time a new drug reaches the market, 12-15 years may have passed. So Congress has devised other ways to extend the lifetime of a patent. Eventually, though, patents will expire and the drug will be the target of competitors.

An interesting side effect of expiring patents is that drug companies, in order to survive, must constantly develop new products. Otherwise, as soon as a patent expires, the company would lose sales to competitors and go out of business.

The National Institutes for Health (NIH) also aids drug and medical device companies by subsidizing research. The NIH budget for 2003 reached $27 billion, a good portion of which is granted to medical researchers at colleges, universities, and medical schools. When the NIH funds research, it is usually directed at a process or study upon which drug and medical device companies can draw to develop their own new products. Sometimes, the research institutions sell or license their discoveries and, thereby, go into partnership with a drug company that develops products from the lab's work.

THE NEXT BIG THING MAY SERVE FEWER, BUT COST MUCH MORE

The drug companies are always searching for the next Big Thing – the drug that generates billions of dollars in sales and, as such, will drive the company's future success. Many new drugs will be targeted at diseases and conditions that serve smaller populations – thousands of people instead of millions. "...[T]hese drugs are more difficult to produce than traditional drugs, which are usually produced by mixing chemical compounds."[19]

The new biotech drugs are often manufactured from live cells in a lab that "looks more like a brewery" than a traditional R&D lab. "Given the complexity of their manufacture and administration, specialty drugs don't become cheaper to make as demand for them grows – the opposite of traditional drugs."[20]

"Avonex, a specialty drug to treat multiple sclerosis, costs more than $1,200 per prescription and specialty drug Enbrel for rheumatoid arthritis is more than $1,100 per prescription..."[21]

Clearly, there is a demand for biotech drugs. No one wants the biotech companies to quit doing research. Many states and cities have created special programs to entice these companies to locate in their towns, seeing it as a great boon for job creation. Still, when a company releases the next wonder drug that costs $10,000 or more per treatment, there will be a public outcry at the cost, and a politician or an editorial writer somewhere will blame Big Pharma.

19. Millie Munshi, "Expensive Drugs Drive Up Health Care Costs," Associated Press, Washingtonpost.com, June 13, 2005.
20. Ibid.
21. Ibid.

Another pricing factor is the realization that once a new product is introduced, a competitor may come out with a similar product long before patent protection expires. The two new drugs will be different, but serve the same purpose. Nexium and Protonix are examples, both of which treat acid reflux. As AstraZenaca prices a new drug like Nexium, it must always consider that Wyeth might produce a new drug like Protonix. It sets the price for Nexium in such a way that it hopes to capture all of its R&D investment, plus profits, and yet, not so expensive that consumers will turn to Protonix to save money.

Drug companies also face the risk that medical science will find other ways to treat or cure a disease. Perhaps a surgeon performs a procedure that stops acid reflux, and therefore, those patients can stop taking Nexium altogether. The patient and surgeon win – AstraZenaca, the drug company, loses.

"In sum, the industry argues that the prices they charge for their products are a reasonable reward for their investment in expensive R&D which ultimately benefits society at large, and that theirs is a high risk industry for which there must be appropriate rewards to induce participation."[22]

Yet, the fact is that no one will buy either drug if they have never heard of it.

GETTING YOU TO BUY

"In 2002, drug manufacturers spent over $19 billion on total product promotion, including samples, brochures, drug detailing (in other words, sales people marketing drugs directly to doctors in their offices), and direct-to-consumer advertising (DTC)..."[23]

---

22. See note 16.
23. See note 11.

That $19 billion includes $12 billion[24] worth of free samples. Doctors pass these out, saving each patient enormous expense. It also gives a doctor time to decide whether to prescribe those medicines permanently. Once those free samples are consumed, the drug companies count on the consumer to buy more...and keep on buying.

Drug companies also buy direct to consumer (DTC) advertising. From 1996, when they spent about $800 million on DTC advertising, overall spending increased to more than $3.3 billion by 2003.[25] Most of those dollars were spent on a few marquee drugs, and tended to be those that treat chronic conditions. For instance, Allegra brings relief to chronic allergy sufferers. Sonofi-Aventis, Allegra's manufacturer, spends hundreds of millions of dollars running TV ads for Allegra. Sonofi-Aventis hopes that those who see their ads will ask their doctor about it.

Some TV ads, like those for lifestyle drugs Viagra or Cialis, promote products that usually are not covered by insurance. Advertising helps to create public demand. McDonald's advertises to get you to their store and sell you a Big Meal Deal. Pfizer advertises Viagra to get you to the pharmacy. Most of us have heard the complaints about TV advertising for these types of drugs that treat men's sexual problems. In fact, many of us blush at them. Yet, they demonstrate something important about the cost of prescription drugs, and the power of advertising.

We are used to seeing drug advertisements, and research shows they work. In fact, just in 1998, "visits to doctors for conditions covered in advertising campaigns rose 263 per cent in the first nine months..."[26] TV ads tell us about wonder drugs that can reduce pain and suffering, make life more enjoyable, and even help us live longer. The

24. Ibid.
25. Ibid.
26. Joan Buckley, "Pharmaceutical Marketing, Time for a Change," *The Electronic Journal of Business and Organizational Studies, Vol. 9, No. 2.*

ads tell us to talk to our doctors, and we do, and doctors respond. Then we suffer sticker shock at the high price of some of those drugs, and hope that our insurance company will pay the bill.

The drug companies know the statistics, and that is why they work hard to get doctors to promote their products. Doctors generate $500,000 a year in fees from seeing patients, but the physician's pen will create $5 million in additional medical expenses, a good share of which are prescription drugs.[27]

Competition helps keep prices from going higher. "According to the National Association of Chain Drug Stores, there are over 35,000 chain drug store pharmacies (for example, CVS), mass merchandiser pharmacies (such as Target), and supermarket pharmacies nationwide."[28] These types of stores fill 60 percent of drug prescriptions. Fighting for their lives are more than 20,000 privately owned "drug stores" and smaller chain stores.

Internet and mail order purchases account for about 13 percent of drug sales. So-called e-pharmacies, companies without fancy buildings that can be located almost anywhere, could provide increasing pressure to hold down future costs.

AND WE BUY THE PRODUCTS

The American Association for Retired Persons (AARP) states, "The biggest driver behind the growth in drug spending, though, is the fact that more people are using more medicines, often the newest and most expensive kinds."[29] And so, "...over half (54 percent) of Ameri-

---

27. Theodore Loftness, M.D., "How Health Care Costs Are Transforming Health Benefits," Slide 18, Medica Broker Forum, Sept. 14, 2005.
28. See note 11.
29. Patricia Barry, "Ads, Promotions Drive Up Drug Costs, Drugmakers Spend Billions Reaching Consumers, Docs," March 2002, aarp.org

cans say they take prescription drugs on a regular basis, and one-fourth (24 percent) say they take three or more drugs regularly. Thirty percent say they currently have more than five prescription drugs in their medicine cabinet."[30] Many insurance plans offer a prescription drug benefit. Most require the insured person to pay a portion of each prescription – $10, $25, $50. The new Medicare Part D insurance is all about making drugs more affordable for seniors. Studies show that those with prescription coverage spend and buy more name brand drugs than those who do not have prescription drug insurance. Insurance insulates them from the true cost of their drugs, and so they spend more. Those without a prescription drug benefit will often buy generic drugs for the simple reason that they cost less, and since these people must pay 100 percent of the cost, they buy the less expensive alternative. This is a great example of how the free market reacts to offset the high cost of innovator drugs.

So, to Answer Your Question

Prescription drugs cost so much because of the incredible expense of developing and marketing new ones. Very few drugs actually make a profit.

There are many alternatives to expensive name brand drugs that people can afford, such as generics and over-the-counter medicines. Still, new name brand drugs will always be in demand, and expensive.

As long as demand remains high and continues to grow – as long as people want relief from pain and suffering, and hope to extend human life – drug companies will continue to manufacture and sell new drugs.

---

30. See note 11.

The high selling price of drugs certainly plays a significant role in the increase of U.S. health care spending. Just as importantly, however, is our passion to consume more of them. Once again, the consumer is insulated from the true cost. We feel entitled to the latest and best drugs, and we consume them because someone else pays the bill – HMOs, health insurance, or the government.

CHAPTER 11
INFANT MORTALITY

Myth: Infant mortality statistics are a good way of measuring the quality of the U.S. health care system.

Truth: Infant mortality statistics depend on how they are collected, who collects them, and for what purpose are they used.

Truth: In third-world nations, infant mortality statistics really do provide a measure of the poor quality of health care services.

Unspoken Secret: 99.7 percent of babies are born alive and will still be living a year later, when they are carried to full term. That is a nearly perfect record.

Why does the United States' infant mortality rate only rank number 17 among the world's modern countries?

Before one can judge the U.S. health care system based on infant mortality, the whole issue must be placed into perspective, because statistics taken out of context usually lead to wrong conclusions.

For instance, you could conclude that Washington, D.C. is too dangerous to visit because it "enjoys" the nation's second highest murder rate.[1] It also lays claim to

1. "Crime Rates for Selected Large Cities, 2002 (offenses known to the police per 100,000 inhabitants)," http://www.infoplease.com/ipa/A0004902.html.

the nation's highest infant mortality (death) rate. In fact, D.C.'s infant mortality rate is nearly twice the national average. From this, you might conclude that no one, adult or unborn child, should go to Washington, D.C., given these grave statistics. Yet, 572,000 people live in the city and hundreds of thousands travel there every day. Isolated statistics don't tell enough of the story.

The U.S. national infant mortality rate is a measure of the average number of infants that die any time during and after delivery up to their first birthday. As of 2000, it stands at 6.9 deaths per thousand.[2] That means that for every 1,000 births, nearly seven babies will die before their first birthday (this does not include fetal deaths – miscarriages, abortions, or the accidental death of a fetus).

The infant mortality rate in Washington, D.C. stood at 13.5 deaths per 1,000 births in 2002, greatly exceeding the national rate.[3] Does this mean that health care for infants in Washington, D.C. far worse than it is in other cities? Are there other factors that affect infant mortality rates that are not related to the health care system?

The issues that directly affect birth and infant mortality rates are numerous. For instance, the infant mortality rate when mothers deliver multiple babies (twins, triplets, etc.) is 31.1 deaths per 1,000 births, a staggering 500% greater than when mothers deliver a single baby. When a single baby is delivered, the U.S. infant mortality rate is 6.1 deaths per 1,000.[4] Looking at this reality without seeing it in context might make us think that we should do everything we can to limit pregnancy to one child at a time, but try telling that to a woman carrying triplets.

Many critics of the U.S. health care system point to our infant mortality rate as a shame and an evidence of failure.

2. "National Vital Statistics Report, Vol 50, No 12," Aug. 28, 2002.
3. Ibid., 10.
4. Ibid., 11.

Singapore enjoys the lowest infant mortality rate of just 2.3 deaths per 1,000.[5] The African nation of Angola is the highest at 193.8.[6] No one would, of course, point to Angola to prove that the U.S. has a great health care system. Neither should they point to Sweden as proof that the U.S. system fails us.

WE FIGHT FOR THE TINIEST BABIES

Not every nation works as hard to keep distressed infants alive as we do. Consider this true story:

> Rumaisa Rahman (born 19 September 2004) is a baby who, according to medical records, is the smallest born baby in history to survive birth after complications due to her size. Rahman was eight inches long and weighed 244 grams (8.6 ounces) [about one-half pound]. She has a twin sister, Hima, also a small baby, weighing just 563 grams (1 pound 4 ounces) at birth.
>
> Rahman was born 25 weeks after gestation. During pregnancy, her mother suffered from pre-eclampsia, making her blood pressure run at high levels. The condition affected Rumaisa the most, putting the baby into distress and leading to birth by caesarean section.
>
> Generally healthy, the twins had to undergo laser eye surgery to correct visual problems, a common occurrence among premature babies. Rahman was tested for cerebral palsy, a worry due to the increased blood pressure of

---

5. "Table 010. Infant Mort Rates & Life Exp at Birth, by Sex," U.S. Census Bureau International Data Base, 1.
6. Ibid., 5.

her mother, but the results indicate that she will not have the disease.

Coincidentally, the hospital where they were born, Loyola University Medical Center in Chicago, Illinois, also delivered the previous record holder for the smallest baby to survive birth, Madeline Mann, who was born in 1989.[7]

At birth, Rumaisa was about the size of a 12 ounce bottle of water. She went home on February 8, 2005 weighing a hefty 5.5 pounds and stretching to 16 inches. Her sister had gone home in December 2004.

At the same time that Rumaisa went home, British doctors reported what they saw as dismal prospects for little British babies like Rumaisa. Their six-year study showed that British babies born very premature often develop serious physical and mental problems as young children. British doctors wondered at the propriety of even allowing such tiny ones to live.

Dr. Eduardo Bancalari, a pediatrician who oversees the care of premature babies at the University of Miami and Jackson Memorial Hospital disagrees with the British doctors' findings. "It's a well-done study, but I don't think it can be applied to what is happening today in the U.S.," he said. Bancalari points out that, "Treatment of premature infants has improved since 1995, when the babies in the [United Kingdom] study were born."[8]

Americans go to heroic lengths to deliver and save tiny babies. In fact, it is not uncommon for a surgeon to perform operations even as complicated as heart surgery on babies

7. Wikipedia, the free encyclopedia online
8. Stephanie Nano, "Premature Babies: Study: 'Miracle babies' have disabilities at age 6, A study in Britain found nearly half of all extremely premature babies had significant disabilities by age 6. Some doubted the study applied to U.S. practices today." Associated Press Writer.

still in the womb.

"It's important to realize that prematurity is a major public health problem. One in eight babies are born prematurely," said Dr. Scott Berns of the March of Dimes.[9]

Dr. Berns knows the true statistics. In the U.S., about 244 babies out of 1,000 born weighing less than 1500 grams (3.4 pounds) will die at birth. Each one of these will be counted against our infant mortality rate. Yet when a U.S. infant weighs at least 2500 grams (5.5 pounds) at birth, and is carried to term, 997 per 1,000 will survive; an infant mortality rate of less than three – nearly perfect![10]

Americans are far more aggressive in their attempts to try to save the lives of tiny premature babies. This aggressiveness lowers the average of our infant survival rate. In many other countries, tiny babies who might have problems surviving, or whose mothers have life-threatening conditions like Rumaisa's mother did, are often aborted. Aborted babies are not counted against the infant mortality rate.

In some of the world's most advanced nations where governments run the health care system, prematurely born infants are viewed as too expensive; it is not cost-effective to allow them to be born. To bring them to the point in life where they can survive outside of a hospital costs hundreds of thousands of dollars, money that could be spent elsewhere. "In the U.S., it is recommended that children be vaccinated against eleven diseases, requiring 20 doses at a cost of about $400 in the public sector..."[11] The $750,000 spent to provide health care for one preemie before that baby can go home could buy a complete vaccination series for 1,875 children.

---

9. Ibid.
10. See note 2.
11. Erica Seiguer, "Who Should Pay for What," Harvard Medical School, 2003.

"In 2001, 12 percent of babies were born prematurely. That was the highest level in 20 years and was due in part to more multiple births, induced labor, and older mothers, who are at higher risk of delivering prematurely."[12] Some of these children develop physical and mental disabilities that require a lifetime of care. A government gatekeeper, the account manager who oversees the health care budget in a single-payer system, could easily calculate that allowing premature babies to be born would rob his budget of tens of millions of dollars. The money spent to help ten children whose health care maintenance would cost $5 million each during a lifetime – $50 million for all 10 – could otherwise be spent providing a full series of vaccinations to almost every one of the 131,530 students in the Detroit, Michigan public school system, or for every one of the 123,500 public school students in the entire state of South Dakota.

Managers of government-run health care systems reason that their job is to care for the masses; spending huge sums of money on a relatively small number of tiny babies might mean that healthy babies with minor health issues will be deprived of medical services. Enough Americans still reject such a brutish form of health care rationing, and will continue to do so as long as we treasure the value of human life.

CULTURAL IMPACT ON INFANT MORTALITY

The health care system gets blamed when babies die at birth. Yet often, the real cause of infant mortality is cultural in nature.

---

12. Jennifer Thomas, "Minor Oxygen Deprivation at Birth Can Dull Mental Skills, Threshold for damage is lower than previously believed, study finds," *HealthScoutNews Reporter,* http://www.hon.ch/News/HSN/511505.html

Thousands of women choose to put off pregnancy until they are nearing 40 or older. Yet, "older women are at an increased risk of pregnancy complications and their infants are more likely to be born with birth defects or low birth weights..." than younger women.[13] Adult women of any age, of course, have a legal right to make a decision to give birth, but it serves to create a distortion in the infant mortality tables.

As a group, Asian-American mothers have the lowest infant mortality; they also give birth at a younger age. The health care system must be prepared to deliver babies to mothers of any age, but when a great number of them are prone to experiencing premature birth, it negatively affects the infant mortality statistics.

Women who are unable to, or have difficulty becoming pregnant seek the aid of a fertility doctor. Yet, "...a rise in use of fertility treatments led to a 400% increase between 1980 and 1998 in the number of multiple births in the United States, according to data released by CDC in December 2003..."[14] Multiple births also correlate to a higher number of infants who die at birth. The cultural decision to have more children, then, negatively affects the infant mortality statistics.

These facts are even more startling:

The infant mortality rate for white U.S. women is 5.7: for African-American women it more than doubles to 13.6.[15] Some people immediately blame racism for this difference, or they blame poverty.

The infant mortality rate for babies weighing less than 1500 grams is 244 per thousand, and the differentiation

---

13. "U.S. Infant Mortality Rate Rises for First time Since 1958, CDC Report Finds," *Across the Nation*, California Health Line, Feb. 12, 2004, http://www.californiahealthline.org/
14. Ibid.
15. See note 2.

based on race is only 10-15 percent. In other words, low-weight, white babies die at a rate just less than low-weight, black babies and almost the same rate as Asian-American babies. *The baby's weight at birth is the most important factor determining his or her chance of survival.*

What causes low birth weight is, however, a critical factor.

Based on the total number of live births, African-American women will deliver low-weight babies at three times the rate of white women. Furthermore, while 2.6 percent of white women who give birth never received prenatal care, that number doubles for African-American women. Confounding this, Asian-Americans, whose infant mortality rate is 4.9 (better than both white and black women) are significantly less likely to seek prenatal care than are whites.

Births to Asian-American mothers under age 20 are more common than are those to whites and African-Americans of the same age. Asian-American mothers also receive less professional prenatal care than African-Americans receive, but have an infant mortality rate 64% below that of African-American women, and 14% below that of white women. Is it possible that in the Asian culture, families provide a good deal of prenatal care, while the same is not true of white and African-American families? Is it likely that close-knit families play a significant role in reducing infant mortality among Asian-American mothers?

The impact of families, and especially two-parent families, is stark when single-parent birth statistics are referenced. During the 1960s, about 17 percent of African-American children were born out of wedlock; today, 22 percent of white children are born out of wedlock. Out-of-wedlock births among African-American women are, however, an astounding 69 percent.[16]

16. See note 2.

Correlation, of course, does not prove cause – but it certainly raises concerns.

Compared to white mothers, African-American women suffer twice the rate of infant mortality, have extremely low-weight babies at a rate 15 percent greater, are twice as likely not to receive prenatal care, and more than two-thirds of their children are born out of wedlock.

What does all this say about the U.S. health care system? Nothing.

What does all this say about the U.S. welfare system that began with the Great Society programs of the 1960s at a time when only 17 percent of African-American women gave birth out of wedlock? What does it say about federal welfare programs that transferred the responsibility for fathers to care for their families to the government? Absolutely everything.

By extension, it seems predictable that if the U.S. decided to aggressively promote the marriage-based, two-parent family across our culture, overall infant mortality rates would drop. The health care system cannot create this kind of norm: it must come from the political and moral will of United States citizens.

CONCLUDING...

We can strive to do better, and in fact, U.S. medical science is always pointed in that direction. Since we are human, we will never achieve perfection – a zero infant mortality rate – but we can try, as long as we are willing to spend whatever it takes to get there.

For babies carried to term, our health care system has reduced infant mortality to about three deaths per 1,000. This is the right way to measure the quality of U.S. health care for moms and their newborn babies.

As for those tiny preemies, U.S. doctors will continue to fight for their lives as long as we hang on to a culture that esteems human life as sacred.

Politicians that use infant mortality to suggest that our health care system is failing us are being dishonest. The social welfare policies they have supported during the last 40 years have negatively impacted illegitimacy rates, as we see that a culture that encourages single-parentage has more to do with infant mortality than does the health care system. To achieve the kind of reductions we all desire in infant mortality means promoting the two-parent, marriage-based family, and that requires political courage of a kind greater than some elected officials are willing to demonstrate.

CHAPTER 12
LIFE EXPECTANCY

Myth: U.S. health care lags behind the modern world as evidenced by shorter life expectancies.

Truth: U.S. life expectancy statistics reflect a complex series of issues not common to other nations.

If we have such a great health care system, why do we die younger than those in 21 other nations?[1] The United States ranks just 22nd in life expectancy, compared to other modern nations. Japan ranks number one.

The life expectancy statistic is a measure of how many years a newborn infant can expect to live. Each year, this statistic is recalculated, and some people believe that it indicates something about the quality of a health care system.

How information is collected and by whom greatly affects the reliability of data, and the conclusions drawn from it. In most areas of the world, government agents assemble the mortality (death) and morbidity (illness and

---

1. Organization for Economic Co-Operation and Development (OECD), Life Expectancy Table for 2003.

disease) data. In many of those nations, the same government that reports health care statistics is also the agency that provides health care services. They have a conflict of interest. Many other nations have no checks and balances to force them to report honest and unbiased statistics. U.S. government information is readily available to anyone who wants it, and scores of private groups analyze and interpret it. This accounts for some of the discrepancies between the U.S. and foreign nations.

Almost non-existent health care systems condemn tens of millions of people to an early death. For instance, Awka, a city of 152,000 people in Anambra State, Nigeria, once had a hospital and medical clinic, but it closed because of government graft and the lack of a stable economy. Unless non-Africans, who are usually religiously motivated or former citizens, come in to provide health care services, many Africans turn to tribal doctors. Their life expectancy is incredibly low, as in Angola, where it is less than 39 years. Nigeria's and Angola's wealthiest citizens, however, receive first class health care by flying to foreign nations, often the U.S., for treatment.

The official life expectancy calculations of many countries, then, are highly suspect. Angolan upper-class citizens may have life expectancies that rival Japan's, which has the longest average life expectancy in the world, while Angolan peasants often may die younger than age 30. Their infant mortality rate is 192.5, among the worst in the world. These factors all serve to distort the Angolan life expectancy statistics. In Angola, however, life expectancy is a factor of class, position, and power.

Since the average U.S. life expectancy lags behind some others, this is counted by some people as proof that our health care system is falling behind, and is even the cause of shorter lives. Some foreign governments, justifying themselves, point to this statistic to show that the U.S. fails in the all-important race to extend life. Since their economies are a fraction of ours, they are unable to afford the broad range of health care services we expect. To keep the people happy, foreign politicians can point to life expectancy statistics in an effort to convince their own citizens that, despite the high level of U.S. health care spending, we are behind them in life expectancy – they have no need to spend more because it makes so little difference.

Unfortunately, some U.S. politicians who favor a government-controlled health care system use these statistics to further their careers. They say we need a radical change. They point out that our life expectancy is behind even tiny nations like Iceland (Iceland ranks number two in the world on the OECD chart, and has a population of less than 300,000). Americans, who seldom hear a rational discussion of this issue, are prone to fall for such rhetoric.

WELL, WHAT ABOUT JAPAN?

Hendrikje "Henny" van Andel-Schipper died peacefully in her sleep in August 2005, at the age of 115. The Dutch woman had this advice for the rest of us: "Keep breathing," and eat pickled herring.

Some foreign health care systems, like Japan's, do seem to produce better results than ours. Chapter 17 explains that system in detail. The Japanese, just like Henny, eat a lot of fish.

Using the OECD tables for 2003, Japan has the longest life expectancy, of 81.8 years (OECD indicates the U.S. life expectancy as 77.2: the National Center for Health Statistics indicates that by 2005, this had become 77.6). On the other hand, Japan's death rate per 1,000 population is greater than in the U.S. (8.8 for Japan, 8.3 for the U.S.)[2] Which of these statistics is more significant? More people die in Japan per 1,000, but those who live, live longer? Statistics can be confusing.

JAPANESE CULTURE, ETHNICITY, AND HEREDITY

There are significant genetic and cultural differences between Japanese and Americans. The United States is known as the "melting pot." Ours is a multi-cultural nation of ethnically diverse people with a rainbow of skin colors stemming from their roots in foreign nations. Interracial and cross-cultural marriages are common. As a result, the U.S. faces genetic and ethnic challenges unlike Japan's.

White Americans comprise about 68 percent of the population, with a growth rate of less than one percent per year. The fastest growing population is among Hispanics, and they comprise the second-largest population group (the

Race	Total Population	Percent of Population	Rate of growth 2000-2004
White	197,325,000	68%	1.2%
Black: African-American	35,577,000	12.3%	4.8%
Hispanic (all sub-groups)	39,340,000	13.6%	17%
Am. Indian & Alaskan Native	2,181,000	.8%	5.2%
Asian	11,667,000	4%	16.5%
Native Hawaiian & Islander	391,000	.13%	8.5%
Two or More Races (Interracial heritage)	3,747,000	1.3%	13.5%

Table 1: United States Population by Racial Groupings[3]

2. "Crude Birth and Death Rates for Selected Countries (per 1,000 population),"
http://www.infoplease.com/ipa/A0004395.html
3. *Abstract of the United States, 2000-2004,* Table 13.

U.S. Census Bureau divides Hispanics into several subgroups). Table 1 shows the racial disparity of the United States.

In contrast, Japan's citizens are 99 percent Japanese, their cultural differences are minimal, and they consume large amounts of fresh fish and fish oil, both of which nutritionists contend contribute to healthier and longer lives. In the U.S., our food preferences are as varied as are our skin colors, running from exotic gourmet and ethnic foods to high fat, mass-produced fast foods. Our weekly diet often includes any or all of these.

These cultural differences become more apparent when we consider Japanese-Americans. Japanese-American men suffer Type II diabetes at rates "…twice as high as comparable samples of men in the U.S. population in general."[4] These Japanese-Americans have been found to consume "…more fat and animal protein than their non-diabetic Nisei counterparts…"[5]

As Japanese adapt to our nitrate-rich salty foods, they seem to have developed "…stomach cancer that is twice as high as most other populations in the U.S."[6] At the same time, as it concerns some other types of major diseases, such as heart ailments or strokes, Japanese-Americans seem to remain healthier than their non-Japanese-American counterparts. The American diet has negatively affected those Japanese who have moved to the United States and adapted their lifestyles to ours.

Unspoken Secret: The Japanese health care system requires individuals to pay a significant portion of their income for health care services, as much as US $4,500 per year, plus insurance premiums that can run as much as

---

4. Marianne K.G. Tannabe, M.D., "Health and Health Care of Japanese-American Elders," Stanford University, 2005. http://www.stanford.edu/group/ethnoger/japanese.html
5. Ibid.
6. Ibid.

another $4,500. In other words, neither a universal nor single-payer, government-gatekeeper health care system is responsible for their longer lives. In fact, the Japanese even must pay for their own vaccinations and normal maternity costs.[7]

The lifespan of different ethnic groups in the U.S. varies greatly. One of the most disturbing statistics is that African-Americans, on average, have a life expectancy of about 5.5 years fewer than U.S. Caucasians. Social scientists and physicians argue over whether such a wide difference is based on hereditary or cultural issues, even forms of discrimination – it may be some or all of these.

AND SO, THE RESULTS ARE...

When all these racial, ethnic, and cultural groupings are averaged out, U.S. life expectancy comes out number 22 among the world's most modern countries.

Canada, with a population of 33 million, ranks eighth in life expectancy. Does that mean that their health care system is better than ours – maybe two or three times better? If average life expectancy is such a critical measurement of the quality of a health care system, it leaves unanswered the question of why thousands of Canadians come to the United States each year to receive critical health care services.

Sweden has a population of fewer than 9 million people. Switzerland's population is 7.5 million, and these two countries have an average life expectancy at 80.3 years. The total population of these two countries is less than 10 different American states. The U.S. population is at 297 million (2005) and growing.

Furthermore, cultural and hereditary factors greatly

---

7. Tomoko Furukawa, "A Primer on Health Care, Health Care Puzzles," *The JapanTimes Online*, Nov. 2004.

influence a society's health. Florida and California are magnets for refugees from some of the world's roughest and unhealthiest nations. Californians often complain about the number of illegal immigrants crossing from Mexico, who use the state's health care system to get treatment not available in their hometowns. Mexicans, by the way, have an average life expectancy of 74.9 years, and when they die younger while in the U.S., they negatively affect our life expectancy rates. When comparing our life expectancy to Japan's, one must ask, "How many illegal immigrants enter and die in Japan?"

Florida attracts millions of retired U.S. residents, as does Arizona. Some health care reformers might point to Florida's higher than average death rate to suggest something is wrong with its health care system. That would ignore the fact that a huge number of older Americans live in the state. Such an analysis, if compared to northern states more heavily populated by younger people, and with a lower death rate, would be absurd. This is, unfortunately, how statistics can be bent for political purposes.

What real conclusions can be drawn from average life expectancy tables as regards the quality of health care? As it applies to modern nations, probably none. As it applies to third world nations, it is obvious.

The life expectancy in Mozambique is 37.1 years. Kenya's is 44.9 years, and in Nigeria it is 50.5 years. Even South Africa, which is a relatively modern nation, has a life expectancy of just 44.2 years.[8] AIDS runs rampant in many parts of Africa, and health care clinics and doctors are almost non-existent in many places.

The African AIDS experience teaches us a very important lesson about how lifestyle choices can and do affect

---

8. "Infant Mortality and Life Expectancy for Selected Countries," 2004, Infoplease.com

life expectancy. Dr. Peter E. Waldron, presidential advisor to Uganda's President Yoweri Museveni, describes the situation:

> Uganda is the AIDS success story because of the President and Mrs. Museveni's strong advocacy for Abstinence before marriage, Be faithful while married, and Condoms for the prostitute and promiscuous. This approach is the famous ABC strategy that attracts the United States religious community toward political support of Uganda, independent of any other evidence of Christian civility. The percentage of the Ugandan population with HIV/AIDS is 5-6 percent.
>
> However, other African nations are not ABC-oriented. Their percentages of population with HIV/AIDS are closer to 40 percent or higher. The primary reason for this extraordinarily high number is promiscuity. Among the poorest of the poor, prostitution is an entry level vocation for survival purposes as parents sell their daughters. Prostitution is common among secondary and university age students for the purpose of raising school fees and day-to-day living expenses.
>
> South Africa presents a bizarre revelation about the exponential explosion of AIDS. It took 10 years to convince the South African president that AIDS was a disease that required education and prevention. Unfortunately, during this slow ignorance response period, witch doctors were advising infected men to have sexual relations with virgins. Sub-

sequently, primary school boys and girls were sexually violated. Today, there are an estimated 4,000,000 men and women with HIV/AIDS in South Africa.[9]

The U.S. does not suffer from this level of sexual promiscuity, but this provides a great example of how lifestyle choice can be a killer. Lifestyle choices are not a reflection of our health care system: they are a moral and cultural issue.

The most honest conclusions to be drawn from life expectancy tables in general are that they reflect complex cultural, hereditary, religious, and political considerations. In many locations, they do not reflect the quality of health care, but the near complete lack of it.

A FEW OTHER THOUGHTS

It is the nature of the U.S. health care system to continue to improve itself. This is due in part to the natural human desire to live longer and healthier lives, and our drive to find new solutions to problems. As such, the health care system will continue to strive to reduce infant mortality and increase life expectancy, as it ought to do. These indexes should continue to improve, unless some disaster befalls America or our government leaders create too many obstacles.

At the same time, there are many factors that influence infant mortality and life expectancy that have absolutely nothing to do with the health care system. These have been mentioned elsewhere, but bear repeating. Clean water, ample power, air conditioning, safe transportation, and

---

9. Commentary provided as a result of the request of the authors. Received via email, Sept. 18, 2005.

effective communications: these all have a profound and direct impact on human life. Natural disasters remind us of these truths. When Hurricane Katrina hit the American Gulf Coast in August of 2005, death came from floods, high winds, and the resultant damage of the storm, not because of the failure of the health care system. We all agree that the death rate was directly related to the slow and ineffective response of local, state, and federal government officials, as well as to the many stubborn people who refused to leave New Orleans.

Consider the ridiculous idea that a government might try to draw conclusions about health care from statistics collected during a time of warfare. What would the infant mortality and life expectancy tables for Japan have looked like in 1945? These had everything to do with the dropping of two atomic bombs and nothing to do with the Japanese health care system.

We cite these examples only to suggest that the very idea that the U.S. infant mortality and life expectancy rankings are a reflection of the quality of health care is absurd. There are more variables at work that lie far beyond the reach of the health care system.

It really is dishonest and immoral for politicians to use infant mortality and life expectancy as wedges to advance their own careers.

CHAPTER 13
THE
UNINSURED "CRISIS"

"Advocates working for the cures of various tragic diseases regularly do the same [lie]. Why not? A little creative lying can draw attention, indignation, and-perhaps most important-the money and political capital to address the actual problem."[1]

Economist Steven D. Levitt

Myth: More than 45 million Americans do not have access to health care because they are uninsured.

Truth: Uninsured Americans do have access to a broad range of health care services at little or no cost to them.

Truth: The number of uninsured Americans is a statistical guess, and is likely far fewer than 45 million, and most likely, 9 to 18 million.

Families USA stated, "Last year's growth in the number of people without health coverage represents the third [annual] increase in a row... escalating from 41.2 million in 2001 to 45 million in 2003."[2]

---

1. Steven D. Levitt and Stephen J. Dubner, *Freakonomics*, William Morrow, 2005, 92.
2. "Census Bureau's Uninsured Number Indicates Third Increase in a Row," FamiliesUSA.org, Aug. 26, 2004.

Other health care advocacy groups, politicians, commentators, health care providers and insurers, have joined together to trumpet these startling numbers. Allowing more than 15 percent of Americans to go without health insurance, they conclude, is wrong and immoral.

Forty-five million uninsured is a great many people, and when more than eight million of those are children, the number seems almost obscene. How could America, such a rich nation, tolerate letting 45 million people go without health care? Well-meaning citizens all across the country ask that question. Health care reform activists make sure we hear the message loud and clear, knowing it appeals to big-hearted, generous Americans.

Surprisingly, some reformers expressed animosity toward the uninsured as First Lady Hillary Clinton once did. "Far from deserving our sympathy, many Americans without health insurance are 'freeloaders,' "[3] Mrs. Clinton said in 1994. She explained that when the uninsured get sick, the rest of us pick up the cost of their care. "It's in our self-interest, she says, to force them and their employers to buy health insurance whether they want to or not."[4]

In 1994, Mrs. Clinton wanted an overhaul of our entire health care system, and one of the linchpins of the legislation she promoted would have forced everyone to buy health insurance. If this had passed, it would seem that 100 percent of Americans would have owned insurance – we will show later that such an assumption is wrong.

Today Mrs. Clinton is a U.S. senator from New York. She still believes that we can no longer stomach having 45 million uninsured. Senator Clinton's idea of mandatory health insurance is gaining steam.

The National Coalition on Health Care, too, strongly

---

3. "Are the Uninsured Freeloaders?" National Center for Policy Analysis, Brief Analysis No. 120, Aug. 10, 1994.
4. Ibid.

promotes the idea of having the government force everyone to buy health insurance. The group claims to be the "nation's largest health coalition" and calls the rate of uninsured "a deepening health care crisis."[5] Their website is awash with statements and statistics about the 45 million or more whom they claim to be uninsured. And they recommend strong action to remedy this "crisis." The most significant of these is "[r]equiring health coverage for all Americans within two to three years after the enactment of legislation."[6] The legislation they refer to here would require everyone to own health insurance.

Those who promote mandatory health insurance want everyone to understand that 45 million uninsured people include many who work for a living. They are not just the sick and poor. Even many middle-class and wealthy persons choose not to buy insurance: to some, that does not seem right.

The idea of mandatory health insurance dates to Germany's first program in 1883. Many foreign nations now require it. During the November 2004 election, Californians just barely defeated a referendum that would have required mandatory health insurance. During the summer of 2005, Republican Massachusetts Gov. Mitt Romney proposed mandatory health insurance. The Minnesota Medical Association, a national leader in health care reform, in 2005 also called for mandatory health insurance. Has the time come when the United States should make mandatory health insurance a federal law?

Certainly, something must be done or 45 million people will continue to suffer needlessly!

Oh?

---

5. "Nation's Largest Health Coalition Calls For Sweeping Changes in Health Care System," National Health Care Coalition, July 20, 2005.
http://www.nchc.org/news/press_releases/2004_07_20.pdf
6. Ibid.

TRIPPING ON THE FACTS

The Employee Benefit Research Institute (EBRI) studied the makeup of the estimate of uninsured persons. EBRI,
"...found two-thirds of spells [time periods] without health
insurance last less than one year, confirming previous
research that..."[7] found the same results. EBRI also found,
"...approximately one-third of all individuals with a spell
of noncoverage [are] chronically uninsured individuals."[8]
These numbers have remained consistent over time. EBRI
believes the number of chronically uninsured American
residents is about 15 million – more like five percent of the
population.

A 2004 study by the Actuarial Research Corporation
(ARC) reported on their investigation of the makeup of the
45 million uninsured, looking at it from several perspec-
tives. It learned some interesting facts about these people.

Some 14 million of the uninsured were eligible to be
enrolled in public insurance programs such as Medicaid or
the SCHIP program for children. In fact, 9 million of the 14
million, "...actually were enrolled in Medicaid during the
year, but were categorized as uninsured in the Census survey."[9] The Census Bureau, which provided the source for
the original claim of 45 million, acknowledged that it had
undercounted those on Medicaid.

"9.3 million uninsured individuals and families earn
$50,000 or more annually and may be able to afford health
insurance. More than half of this group – 4.8 million people – earn more than $75,000 per year."[10]

$50,000 a year is greater than the average American

7. Craig Copeland, "Characteristics of the Nonelderly with Selected Sources of Health
Insurance and Lengths of Uninsured Spells," EBRI Issue Brief No. 198, June 1998,
Employee Benefit Research Institute, Washington, D.C.
8. Ibid., 1.
9. *The Uninsured in America*, Blue Cross, Blue Shield Foundation, 2005, 4.
10. Ibid, 6.

family income of around $44,000. $75,000 places a family near the upper middle class. There may be health or credit reasons why some of these are uninsured, but it is likely a good number of them just choose not to buy insurance. The cost of insuring mom, dad, and two children with a good $1,500 deductible policy is about $380 a month, which seems affordable for a $75,000 income family – or even a $50,000 income family – if they had the will to purchase it. (In some states, families with incomes larger than $50,000 can receive Medicaid or tap into other subsidized health insurance programs.)

Many young people are willing to bet that they will stay healthy so they choose to be uninsured. People younger than 35 make up 26 percent of the American population, but more than 45 percent of the uninsured.[11] That 21 year-old without health insurance would pay about $100 a month for a $1,500 deductible policy with a $3 million lifetime benefit. The fact that they exercise this choice frustrates many health care reformers, like Senator Clinton, because these are the ones who become "freeloaders" if they get sick.

ARC identified 23 million persons who either really are insured in a tax-subsidized program, or have chosen not to be insured. This shrinks the 45 million closer to 22 million uninsured.

Who are the 22 million?

ARC reports that 22 million of the uninsured earn less than $50,000 a year and they may have trouble affording insurance. "Some may be between jobs or recent college graduates who decide to go without coverage, or they work for firms that don't offer health benefits. Others cannot afford health care insurance because they are unemployed or don't earn enough to pay for coverage on their own."[12]

---

11. Ibid, 13.
12. Ibid, 8.

Some people, like those just out of college, are caught in a temporary time warp between graduation and their first real job. They are enjoying the healthiest time of their lives and see no need to spend money for insurance.

A segment of the population refuses to take care of itself no matter the cost. They will never buy health insurance even if the law requires it.

There remains some unknown number of people who want health insurance but really cannot afford it.

Some 47 percent of the uninsured either work in small businesses, or their parents do. "Low-wage workers in small firms are far more likely to lack coverage than other workers. A good number of these are part-time workers. Sixty-four percent of low-wage workers in firms with fewer than 10 employees lack employer coverage. Firms with fewer than 10 employees have the highest overall uninsured rate, regardless of worker income level."[13]

Small companies are often cash-strapped and marginally profitable, meaning it is difficult for them to offer employee health insurance benefits. Employees must purchase coverage on their own, or go without. In some cases, they would be covered by their spouse's health insurance. Forcing these small employers to buy group health insurance could make the difference between staying in business and closing their doors.

African-Americans and Hispanics make up about 28 percent of the non-elderly population but represent 42 percent of the uninsured.

Almost 33 percent of the uninsured are Hispanics, many of whom recently came from countries that had national health care systems. Some of these may qualify for Medicaid but are illegal immigrants and so, to avoid being arrested and deported, they fear signing up.

---

13. Ibid, 11.

Investor's Business Daily estimates that there are as many as 11 million illegal immigrants in America. The total number of illegal immigrants who receive free or subsidized health care services is unknown. What is known is that providing health care for illegal immigrants is expensive, and taxpayers bear the costs. "Last year...[Los Angeles] County spent $340 million to treat uninsured patients, and the state was hit with $1.4 billion in non-reimbursed health care costs. Texas spent $850 million, and Arizona, $400 million."[14] In contrast, Canada and France, with their government-run systems, only provides health insurance coverage to legal residents.

Another 6 million of the 45 million uninsured go without coverage for only a few months. Most of these 6 million owned health insurance for most of the year.[15]

THE TRULY UNINSURED – WHY IS IT IMPORTANT?

So, really, who are the uninsured? "The bottom line: About 8.2 million Americans, not 45 million, are chronically uninsured and low income. And they are the working poor. They have jobs but, because of the high cost of insurance, no coverage,"[16] wrote economist David Gratzer.

Devon Herrick, of the National Center for Policy Analysis, suggested a different number of uninsured: "...those too rich for Medicaid but too poor to afford insurance is close to 18 million people."[17]

Despite these more realistic numbers, many health care reformers, like the National Coalition for Health Care,

14. Jim Meyers, "Illegals: The Real Cause of Health Insurance Crisis," *NewsMax.com*, May 2, 2005.
15. David Gratzer, "What Health Insurance Crisis?". *The Los Angeles Times,* Aug. 29, 2004.
16. Ibid.
17. Andrew Damstedt, "Analysts suggest mandatory health coverage," *The Washington Times*, May 5, 2005.

cling to the 45 million number as they demand that the federal government pass a law mandating that everyone own health insurance. If, of course, more than 15 percent of the population really does go without access to health care (or even health insurance), such an argument might seem prudent, even though it violates America's cherished notion of freedom of choice. At 3-6 percent, the real index of the hardcore uninsured, the argument is far more difficult to make.

Mandating health insurance for everyone would create a new bureaucratic system far larger than Social Security and Medicare, and a tax increase per month of hundreds of dollars for each family. The experience of foreign nations that have mandatory health insurance proves that total health care spending would go up, not down (see chapter 14). Insurance premiums would rise, not fall. Millions of individuals would be stripped of their freedom to spend their own money as they see fit. Yet, many still ask, "Isn't this better than having them go without health care?"

Jon Gabel, of the Health Research and Educational Trust, said, "The quality of care uninsured patients receive also is less than that given to insured patients. He said the uninsured enter the hospital sicker, are discharged sooner, and are more likely to die in the hospital."[18]

Gabel raises another question for America's citizens. In a country where individual initiative and hard work are respected, where employees can choose to spend their money as they please, must we provide equal health care services for everyone? Is health care a right that falls into what the Declaration of Independence calls the inalienable right to "life, liberty and the pursuit of happiness"?

President George W. Bush passionately promotes the

18. Ibid.

"culture of life" argument. He believes that all humans should have the right to life until the natural occurrence of death.

THE FAIRNESS DOCTRINE

We need to step aside for a moment and address the issue of "fairness." In the health care debate, fairness has become a doctrine. The fairness doctrine is the idea that everyone is entitled to the same outcomes, no matter their circumstances. For instance, in a 100-yard dash between a college track star and a 60-year old man, to achieve fairness, the old man gets a 60-yard head start, giving him a fair chance to win the race. To make a test fair for women, a fire department reduces the weight which a candidate must carry so that a proper proportion of females can pass the test. Admission standards are set lower for some categories of students so that they have a fair chance to enter college.

As it touches health care, fairness means that everyone, regardless of income, job status, location, personal responsibility, or any other factor, must have access to an affordable and equal quality of health care. Fairness demands that such a system must follow one pattern that fits all. This ignores reality. Some people work hard to preserve their health, while others abuse themselves with drugs, alcohol, tobacco, laziness, and poor diet. Fairness also places "high needs" patients in jeopardy – disabled, elderly, chronically ill, and sick babies – simply because they consume more services, and what they consume is often very sophisticated and expensive.

Equal access denies reality. Nothing is equal. Two surgeons operating in adjoining rooms in the same hospital, trained the same way, are not equal. Even the same surgeon, operating on two different persons on the same day in the same room might provide unequal skills to the second patient. Hospitals that cater to more chronically ill patients may be judged as offering "unfair" health care if compared to a new facility located in a suburb populated by healthy citizens.

Health care does not lend itself well to an assembly-line mentality where everything that comes out the door is identical.

The only way to create a truly "fair" health care system is to offer one doctor, one hospital, and one clinic for everyone; a system that would result in massively long lines in which patients would die while waiting.

The debate about promoting a culture of life as opposed to a perceived quality of life rages on, and directly effects health care costs. Those who, like President Bush, believe all human life – unborn, disabled, comatose, vegetative – is sacred, need to recognize that their beliefs cost money. Those who believe that human life should be determined by a value judgment based on quality, will have to recognize that if they make powerful government the arbiter of life, it will lead to sliding down the slope to discriminating against our most vulnerable citizens – sick, aged, and disabled persons.

WHAT IF THE LAW MANDATED THAT EVERYONE MUST OWN HEALTH INSURANCE?

The best estimate of the number of hard-core uninsured is between 9.3 and 18 million – somewhere between 3-6 percent of the U.S. population.

A broad-based coalition of organizations and politicians[19] advocate for mandatory health insurance for everyone. They do this because they believe that people going without insurance deprives them of health care and drives up its costs for all the rest of us. To make their point that mandatory insurance is essential, they suggest that "45 million" uninsured Americans cannot receive adequate health care. They equate owning health insurance with receiving health care. This strikes them as unfair.

A consistent human trait is that we do not always comply with laws. In some cases, the sheer number of persons breaking a law sends a specific message: the law is unfair and unenforceable, and that it does not have citizens' support. Mandating insurance is like this.

Many states mandate that all auto owners must own car insurance, yet a large number refuse. Jim Genetti, an Idaho transportation official, wrote, "I have seen statistics showing that about 30% of all Idaho drivers are without insurance..."[20] even though Idaho law requires it.

Minnesota mandates auto insurance and it is a no-fault state. According to the Insurance Federation of Minnesota, one out of six – almost 17 percent – of Minnesota drivers refuse to buy auto insurance. That number exceeds even the highest national estimate of those who go without health insurance.

Wisconsin does not mandate auto insurance. Of 208,000 accidents reported during 2003, "75% of the vehicles were insured, 12.6% were uninsured and 11.6% were unknown."[21]

---

19. Minnesota Medical Association, Gov. Mitt Romney and the Massachusetts Assembly, 100 members of the House in the 103rd. Congress, National Coalition on Health Care and their long list of supporters and members (including three former US Presidents), and many more.

20. Mr. Genetti responded to a personal email sent to him by author Dave Racer on May 12, 2005. Mr. Racer had asked Mr. Genetti what the estimate of uninsured motorists might be in Idaho.

21. Email received on May 13, 2005, from DOT-DMV Traf-Acc-Sec (traf-acc-sec.dmv@dot.state.wi.us).

Evidence suggests that mandatory no-fault auto insurance has driven up the costs of insurance, rather than reduce costs.

At the time of our writing, Hawaii remained the only U.S. state to have a mandatory health insurance law, in place since 1974. In Hawaii, "Employers must provide health care coverage to employees who work at least twenty (20) hours per week..."[22] and meet other income standards. Unfortunately, Hawaii officials have no way of knowing how many employers are actually complying with the law, because it does not collect those statistics. Noreen Ichikawa, the health chief in the Hawaii Department of Labor, said that the department has begun random checks of employers and hopes to root out those who cheat. Ichikawa suggested that both employers and employees play games with the government to avoid paying the insurance costs.

In 2002, despite its mandatory insurance law, Hawaii's uninsured rate stood at 10 percent, after having ballooned to nearly 30 percent in the 1990s. That 10 percent number greatly exceeds the 3-6 percent of Americans who are chronically uninsured, even though Hawaii mandates employers to enroll all workers.

If reformers succeed in passing national or state laws mandating that all citizens must purchase health insurance, many millions of employers and employees will try to find ways around the law, choosing to go without insurance. As many as 10 percent or more Americans will remain uninsured even if insurance becomes mandatory (mirroring the experience of foreign nations and Hawaii).

Mandatory health insurance will drive up health care spending and the costs of insurance for everyone for several reasons. The primary reason is the perception that health

---

22. Prepaid Health Care Act, http://www.hawaii.gov/labor/ded/aboutphc.shtml.

care is now nearly free. Armed with an insurance policy, previously uninsured Americans would go to the doctor more often: Medicare and Medicaid taught us this lesson. More health care consumption (demand) always increases costs for everyone (supply). Meanwhile, hardcore non-conformists will still refuse to buy or sign up for insurance. A governmental agency will be tasked with policing us to ensure compliance, and another agency will need to collect unpaid premiums. Whether this would fall to the IRS or a new agency is unknown, but someone will have to enforce such a law.

As a result of mandating health insurance, health care spending would surely go up once again.

WHAT KIND OF HEALTH CARE CAN THE UNINSURED ACCESS?

With all the talk about providing health insurance for uninsured U.S. residents, one might believe that they do not receive any health care services. Federal law requires that all hospital emergency rooms accept everyone who walks through the door, and health care reformers rightly claim that this is a bad way to provide care to the uninsured. They ignore a multitude of other programs available to our poorest citizens. The government has created scores of programs to meet the needs of the uninsured, or find insurance for them. Millions of people use them every year. InsureKidsNow.gov says, "Now, you may have one less thing to worry about. Your state, and every state in the nation, has a health insurance program for infants, children and teens."[23]

Lower-income parents, and even many middle-income families, really have no excuse for not securing insurance

23. Insure Kids Now, http://www.insurekidsnow.gov/

for their children – they very nearly have to choose otherwise, or have to show no interest in learning about the number of plans available to them at little or no cost. The programs are there to be used, and taxpayers already are spending billions of dollars on them.

The authors wanted to know how much money the federal government spends on health care for the poor and uninsured. Coming up with such a number is difficult. It includes direct subsidies, federal grants for programs, funding for buildings and equipment, and money for educating medical professionals. Other funds are spent on medical research, regulation, and enforcement, a part of which can be directly or indirectly related to the cost of providing free or reduced cost programs to uninsured Americans.

As for free care, the authors wrote to the United States Health Resources Services Administration (HRSA) on April 15, 2005, asking, "We would like to know what the per capita value of free care was in the latest year for which data is available. Is there any calculation as to the foregone fees that would otherwise have been charged by health care providers if those patients could have paid their own bills, or had insurance to do so?"

This free care is a result of health care providers using federal government funds released under the 1946 Hill-Burton Act. That law provides funds to medical facilities.

"In fiscal year 2003, the approximately 100 facilities obligated under the standard Hill-Burton regulations provided $16,783,212 in uncompensated services at allowable credit. (The allowable credit is a calculation which converts the amount a facility charges for services to a cost basis.) This amount does not include the uncompensated services provided by the approximately 235 facilities certified under one of our compliance alternatives, e.g., public facility compliance alternative."[24]

The American Hospital Association estimates that in 2003 it gave away $24.9 billion in uncompensated care, about 5.5 percent of its members' total billings.[25]

Almost 65 percent of American doctors donated an average of 7.5 hours a week of care, valued at more than $58,180 each annually.[26] We know that there are about 800,000 doctors in America today. If just 60 percent of them donated an average of $50,000 care each year, that would be worth $24 billion.

Some $1.8 billion in federal tax dollars flowed to community health centers during 2005. These programs grew out of President Lyndon Johnson's "War on Poverty" during the mid-1960s. "...[I]t was the passage of the landmark Economic Opportunity Act of 1964 that marked the birth of America's Community Health Centers [CHCs]. The health center model that emerged targeted the roots of poverty by combining the resources of local communities with federal funds to establish neighborhood clinics in both rural and urban areas around America."[27]

To find the clinic nearest you, or just to see for yourself how extensive these tax-subsidized services are, go to http://ask.hrsa.gov/pc/. There you can input a zip code and find the clinic nearest you.

CHCs' creators envisioned that these centers would "provide accessible, affordable personal health care services to low-income families."[28] They wanted to serve the needs of uninsured and underinsured persons. The "unin-

---

24. DFCRCOMM (HRSA), April 19, 2005, in an email to Mr. Racer, responding to his question.
25. "Health Forum," Annual Survey, (1990-2003), American Hospital Association.
26. 2001 American Medical Association Patient Care Physician Survey.
27. "About Health Centers, History of Community Health Centers," National Association of Community Health Centers, http://www.nache.com/about/aboutcenters.asp.
28. Bureau of Primary Health Care, http://bphc.hrsa.gov/programs/CHCPrograminfo.asp

sured and underinsured" is the same group of people that modern reformers wish to provide with health insurance. Free and subsidized care, according to them, is not good enough.

The CHCs have established themselves in communities across the country. They have won funding from many sources, including Medicaid, Medicare, and other state-sponsored programs for low-income persons. "...[H]ealth centers on average receive only 26% of their total revenue from federal grants. The largest single source of revenue is Medicaid, representing 36% of total revenue and 64% of all patient-related revenue. Another major source (13%) of revenue comes from non-federal grants and contracts, the vast majority of which comes from state and local funds."[29] The CHCs have built an extensive state and national matrix of support and training programs to carry on their work, and one would presume that the costs of this support comes from the same funding sources as does the care they provide to indigents.

President George W. Bush has joined previous presidents since Lyndon Johnson by urging Congress to expand funding of these programs. "In 2002, the President launched an initiative to expand access to health care by creating 1,200 new or expanded health center sites and serving an additional 6.1 million people by 2006."[30]

The budget for community health center programs during 2005 grew more than $200 million to $1.8 billion. The 2005 budget will allow the programs to be extended to 15 million Americans in 3,800 locations across the nation, at the rate of about $120 per year for each person served. About 7 million of these people live in rural areas. If historic averages continue, about 6 million uninsured persons

---

29. See note 27.
30. "FY 2005 Budget in Brief," Health Resources and Services Administration, http://www.hhs.gov/budget/05budget/healthres.html#ex

will receive their primary health care at one of these 3,800 clinics.

Are these CHCs doing an acceptable and decent job? "Studies have found that the quality of care provided at health centers is equal to or greater than the quality of care provided elsewhere. Moreover, 99% of surveyed patients report that they were satisfied with the care they receive at health centers."[31]

CHCs seem to be meeting many of the needs of low-income, uninsured, and underinsured Americans, and they are doing a great job of it.

STILL OTHER CATEGORIES OF ASSISTANCE FOR UNINSURED PEOPLE

Another segment of uninsured persons live with AIDS or are HIV infected. "The FY 2005 budget requests <u>$2.1 billion</u> for the ... HIV/AIDS program, a net increase of $35 million over FY [fiscal year] 2004." This program "...provides services to approximately 530,000 individuals each year with little or no insurance."[32] [Emphasis in the original] The average spent on each HIV/AIDS infected person is $3,962 per year.

Special programs have also been established to help pregnant women and children, and these go beyond the State Children's Health Insurance Program (SCHIP) that provides for children's health needs. "The budget requests $730 million for the Maternal and Child Health (MCH) Block Grant..."[33] MCH provides services to 27 million women and their children – about $27 per capita. The government does not disclose how many of these are unin-

---

31. See note 27, 4.
32. See note 30, 4.
33. Ibid., 5.

sured, though it is likely many would be, or at least, be underinsured.

To receive an MCH block grant, states have to promise to spend some of their own money on acceptable programs. "States match $3 in funds for every $4 in Federal funds they receive."[34] This federal/state partnership developed into more than $3 billion in spending to "meet critical challenges in maternal and child health..."[35] Many States overmatch the federal funds. To overmatch means that the states actually spend more than federal law requires.

Another federal program pays $278 million for family planning services. Again, no estimate is given as to how much of this money goes to pay the costs of uninsured patients.

Since 1985, all hospital emergency rooms in facilities that accept Medicare patients are required by law to treat anyone despite their ability to pay. While this is certainly not the ideal way to treat a person with a chronic problem, or who simply has the flu or a bad cold, it is the ultimate safety net for a person without insurance.

Chapter nine discussed Medicaid. It is the largest single health care program for low-income and uninsured persons, already serving more than 36 million persons.

AMERICANS ARE GENEROUS AS THEY HELP OTHERS WITH HEALTH CARE NEEDS

Alongside these federally funded clinics stand unknown numbers of charitable health care providers. The value of their services are likely impossible to quantify.

Gospel Rescue Missions, like the one in St. Paul, Minnesota, are equipped with dental and health clinics that minister to the needs of some of America's most difficult

---

34. "Maternal and Child Health Bureau," http://www.hrsa.gov/annualreport/part5.htm.
35. Ibid.

cases. Mission workers refer those who need more extensive service to a nearby community health center, or to Regions Hospital, a facility that has provided tax-supported and charity care since 1872.

Indigent people of all faiths facing death can receive high-quality, loving and tender hospice care at Our Lady of Good Counsel Homes in Atlanta, New York, Philadelphia, or St. Paul. Our Lady of Good Counsel Homes refuse to charge anything for their services.

First Baptist Church in Leesburg, Florida, a small city of 17,000 residents, is a shining example of how people of goodwill offer low-cost or free health care for hurting people. The church operates a "Ministry Village" that sits adjacent to their church campus. The village, open to anyone in need, includes a Benevolence Center, Children's Shelter Home, Teen Shelter Home, Pregnancy Care Center, a Men's Residence, Women's Care Center, and a Community Medical Care Center.

The Shriners' Hospitals are famous for their free care for children with some of the most serious diseases. They also fund millions of dollars in research to eliminate chronic health problems.

These are but a few examples of charitable medical service providers available to uninsured persons in locations all across the U.S.

Charities dedicated to wiping out certain diseases raise hundreds of millions of dollars every year. By allowing taxpayers to deduct contributions, governments have formed a funding partnership with them, but they are on their own as it concerns raising and spending their funds.

You may know someone who cannot afford necessary drugs. There are at least three ways that Americans have provided help. First, a person may purchase generic drugs, which cost as little as 26 percent of their name brand counterparts. Secondly, over-the-counter drugs and medicines provide inexpensive relief. Thirdly, help is offered at http://www.PPARX.org, a website that helps low-income people locate a place to find affordable drugs. Drug companies also promote free and low-cost programs for their name brand drugs.

The authors recognize that they have mentioned only a tiny number of America's great charitable health care institutions, and even by mentioning them, they know they have offended those whose names were left out of this book. They did this without meaning to slight any organization or ministry. Those about which they wrote are merely offered as examples of the vast amount of free and subsidized health care available to America's uninsured persons. The authors are concerned that reformers, in their zeal, will do damage to such institutions as governments impose ever-increasing requirements on them and, as happened to some extent in Germany, perhaps force them out of business. That would be a tragic mistake.

SOME BASIC CONCLUSIONS

At the beginning of this section we stated, "Estimates from numerous sources, including the U.S. Census Bureau, state that at least 45 million Americans are uninsured, meaning they are without health insurance. Doesn't this indicate that our health care system has a serious weakness? Doesn't this mean that tens of millions of people are going without health care, and isn't that unfair?"

First, the discussion should begin with the true number of uninsured persons, and not exaggerate the problem so as to create a crisis that only politicians can solve. If they were honest about this, we could find better ways of serving the needs of those who fall through the cracks.

Secondly, we know that America really does have a persistent problem with hardcore uninsured persons, perhaps 3-6 percent of the population. This is not proof of a weakness in a market-based health care system. It is a problem that our system addresses through a multitude of subsidized health care programs.

Thirdly, Americans continue to invest billions of dollars and volunteer hundreds of millions of hours to provide health care services for our poorest and most vulnerable persons. Sometimes, it is true, these services may be less easily accessible than those received by insured Americans. No matter what reforms we adopt, we must be careful not to disrupt or destroy the good work of our charitable health care providers.

The authors agree that health care funding needs reform, and that the system should constantly be improved, but not because of a mythical "crisis" of 45 million uninsured Americans.

Many U.S. health care reformers praise foreign health care delivery systems. They trumpet universal coverage, equal access, less national spending, and high-quality care, even for their poorest citizens.

Before anyone jumps on the single-payer, foreign health care system bandwagon, however, they had better read in the next section what we discovered when we took a closer look.

CHAPTER 14
LOOKING ABROAD
FOR A CURE

Question: Aren't there many health care systems in the world that are superior to ours? Shouldn't we be reforming our system to look like theirs, or at least choose from the best features of each one to reform ours?

To answer this question, we look to these five countries: Canada, the United Kingdom (England and Northern Ireland), Japan, France, and Germany. We chose Canada because it is a pure, single-payer system. We chose the United Kingdom and Germany because their systems are popular among U.S. reformers, and Germany's system is the most mature. We chose France because it is often ranked number one in the world. And we chose Japan, because it is the nation with the longest life expectancy.

We discovered that each of these systems shares common problems with us. Costs are rising, people want more, populations are aging, and technology keeps sending costs higher. We found that it is universally true that people everywhere want others to help pay their health care bills.

In each of these five major countries, the national government sets health care policy and controls pricing. In four of these countries, government commissions and bureaucrats micromanage health care for their residents - they are the health care gatekeepers. They control the gate by determining what kind and how much health care people receive, who will pay for it, and how much it will cost. In these countries, the central government holds monopoly control over health care.

A monopoly means limiting or eliminating all competition. The monopolist controls everything. America's founding fathers knew that monopolies meant mischief, and were to be vigorously opposed. So in the United States, Congress has made monopolies illegal, and the courts have agreed. Our founding fathers even opposed too much monopoly power centered in the government. As a result, in the United States, the free market still provides the bulk of health care, although governments pay 46 percent of its cost.

Many U.S. health care reformers passionately support a government-controlled, single-payer system; granting the U.S. government monopoly power over health care. They believe that it would give every American access to affordable and equal health care, without regard to income, health, or location. They see that a single-payer plan "makes it possible to place a large part of the country's [health care] revenues in a single state [federal government] fund and to allocate them for..."[1] a national health plan to provide equal care to everyone.

A U.S. single-payer system, then, would be a federal system, administered from Washington, D.C. This would be a socialist approach to health care. "Socialism is a system of philosophy which requires that the whole machinery of production and distribution of goods and services shall be owned, controlled, and operated, not by individu-

---

1. "Soviet Ownership," Great Soviet Encyclopedia, 1975, 241.

als and competitive forces in the interests of a few, but by society in a cooperative manner for the advantage of all."[2] Furthermore, "Socialism is at once a criticism of the existing order, a philosophy of social progress, a conception of an ideal society, and a definite movement for social reorganization."[3] Advocates for a single-payer health care system, whether purposefully or not, reveal that they prefer a complete reorganization of our economy and society. They prefer a strong, central government to individual freedom and choice, monopoly to competition.

Distinct from a socialist approach to providing health care is to enable the free enterprise system to flourish. Free enterprise is "...an economic and political doctrine holding that a capitalist economy can regulate itself in a freely competitive market through the relationship of supply and demand with a minimum of governmental intervention and regulation."[4]

The U.S. health care system today is a blend of socialism – Medicare, Medicaid and other state-based programs – and free enterprise, using private insurance and personal out-of-pocket payments for services. Services are delivered by a mixture of private for-profit and non-profit, charitable, and public health care providers.

During the past 40 years, federal and state governments have asserted themselves at an increasing pace into the health care marketplace. This has made it more difficult for the system to take full advantage of competition, although many insurance companies and medical providers do compete for our business. Most certainly, the mixing of central government regulation with the free market has driven up health care costs, and brought us to the point where politicians now talk about taking us all the way to a

---

2. Gordon S. Watkins, *An Introduction to the Study of Labor Problems,* Thomas Crowell Company, 1922, 556-557.
3. Ibid., 557.
4. Definition of Free Enterprise, Infoplease.com

socialist, single-payer system.

Yet, at the same time that we talk about moving toward the socialist health care models of foreign countries, they are moving toward our free market system. "Ironically, over the course of the past decade almost every European country with a national health care system has introduced market-oriented reforms and turned to the private sector to reduce health costs and increase the value, availability, and effectiveness of treatments. In making such changes, more often than not those countries looked to the United States for guidance."[5]

U.S. SPENDING INCREASES LESS THAN GERMANY AND JAPAN – SAME AS UNITED KINGDOM

The U.S. health care system differs greatly from others because there still remains vigorous economic competition among providers and payers. As well, the United States offers an abundance of health care services and products not common everywhere else, and we spend more. During 2003, U.S. citizens paid about 14 percent of their health care costs out of pocket while private insurance companies paid about 36 percent. Various government units paid 46 percent. A host of different sources accounted for the remaining four percent.[6] That same year, the U.S. spent $1.7 trillion on health care, 15.3 percent of our GDP.

The central reason that we spent $1.7 trillion is because we have the world's most powerful, most successful economy. Remarkably, we spent this money during a time when the economy was just barely recovering from a recession.

5. John C. Goodman, "Health Care in a Free Society, Rebutting the Myths of National Health Insurance," National Center for Policy Analysis, Dallas, TX, Jan. 27, 2005, 2.
6. "Table 1: National Health Expenditures, Aggregate and Per Capita Amounts, Percent Distribution, and Average Annual Percent Growth, by Source of Funds: Selected Calendar Years 1998-2003," Centers for Medicare and Medicaid, U.S. Government.

In fact, it is very likely that one of the reasons the American economy has regained so much strength since 2001 is due to the millions of high-paying health care jobs.

Most foreign nations, able to show health care spending far below ours, are unable to spend any more than they do because of their smaller GDP, and because their citizens will not tolerate increased taxes. They do not have the discretionary income necessary to support a larger system. Unlike in the United States where people can freely spend their own money on additional health care services if they choose, in some countries, it is illegal for people to purchase health care services with their own money.

Before we look at these foreign health care systems, let's look at total spending on health care and other related factors in Table 1 on the next page.

U.S. residents spend, on average, $2,576 more per year, per person on health care than Germans do, the next highest spending nation. Our $1.7 trillion in health care spending nearly exceeds the entire Gross Domestic Product of France or the United Kingdom, and far exceeds that of Canada. Japan's economy produces a significant GDP, but they still spend only half of what we do per person for health care. In the U.S., our hard work, economic success, and level of discretionary spending make it possible for us to afford greater health care spending.

Even though in these five foreign countries, governments play a central role in health care, they struggle to control increases in total spending. The United Kingdom's health care costs have risen at the same rate as ours, but Germany and Japan have seen more rapid increases. Only Canada, with its severely strict single-payer health care system and global budgets, has managed to hold their increases to an almost insignificant level.

Total Spending on Health Care and Other Related Factors: Six Countries

Country	Population[8]	Gross Domestic Product (GDP)[7]	$ Spent on Health Care	% of GDP[9]	Per Capita	Increase 1990-2003
United States	296 million	$11.0 trillion[10]	$1.7 Trillion	15.3	$5,743	28%
Germany	82 million	$2.36 trillion	$260 billion	11.1	$3,170	30.5%
France	61 million	$1.74 trillion	$176 billion	10.1	$2,885	17.4%
Canada	33 million	$1.02 trillion	$101 billion	9.9	$3,060	10%
Japan	127 million	$3.7 trillion	$366 billion	7.9	$2,882	33%
United Kingdom (England)	60 million	$1.78 trillion	$137 billion	7.7	$2,283	28%

7. "Economic Statistics by Country, 2004," Infoplease.com
8. "Area and Population of Countries, Mid-2005 Estimates," Infoplease.com
9. "Total Expenditures on Health-% of gross domestic product," OECD, 2003.
10. This citation differs from the data in note 7, and instead, reflects the data in Table 1 of note 6. This was done to provide the same data used throughout the book, when two sources differ. We use the U.S. Government figures.

204

OVERVIEW

As we studied these five health care systems, we discovered a cycle. First, they start with a strict, centrally-controlled monopoly system, where the federal government controls every aspect of health care, and individuals are not allowed freedom to use their own money for additional services. Eventually, demand for services and the money available to provide them collide head on, and the system hits a plateau. Once at that plateau, the people begin to demand more than the government can deliver.

Eventually, on a limited basis the people win the right to spend their own money to get better or more services, and the system takes tiny steps toward free market reforms. As people are free to use their own money, it causes a spike in health care spending (as in Germany, Japan and the UK). The governments, alarmed by these increases, try to assert more controls and bring services and spending back into what the government views as balanced. The people, however, will never be satisfied with what the government can provide. The United Kingdom's National Health Service states, "We shall never have all we need...Expectations will always exceed capacity."[11]

Every one of these countries suffers from high utilization. In four of them, people use health care services liberally because they appear to be free or nearly free. Since their out-of-pocket expenses are limited – or none – they have no reason not to keep going to the doctor. They have little or no personal financial risk, and the high taxes they pay makes them feel entitled to use the services.

Canada is a relatively immature socialized system and is caught in an ongoing struggle to maintain its socialist

---

11. "The NHS from 1948-1957," http://www.nhs.uk/England/AboutTheNhsHistory/1948-1957.cmsx

roots. It still clings tightly to its global budgets and the contemptuous complaints of the sick people it leaves in long waiting lines.

CHAPTER 15
LOOKING NORTH:
CANADIAN HEALTH CARE

Canada's 33 million citizens live in a country of 3.86 million square miles, slightly larger than the United States. Canada spends $101 billion, 9.9 percent of its $1.02 trillion GDP on health care.

Many U.S. reformers point to Canada's socialist health care system as the best model, asserting that it is free, provides equal access and benefits, is fair and doesn't discriminate, and has controlled health care spending.

The reason it is called socialistic is because Canadian health care is delivered by a single-payer system that is controlled by the national government. Provincial governments administer the programs, but the federal government controls the money and sets health care policy. The same system in the U.S. would mean that Washington, D.C. would set all health care policy, control the supply of doctors and hospitals, collect all the money, and then send it to the 50 states to administer the programs it approves.

"Health Canada plays five core roles in order to realize our vision...to help us and others make informed, effective choices...[as] Leader/Partner, Funder, Guardian/Regulator,

Service Provider, Information Provider."[1] (Health Canada is the name of the Canadian system.) The Minister of Health is in charge of the national health system.

The Canadian health care plan is anchored by its commitment to these principles: "Prevent and reduce risks to individual health and the overall environment; promote healthier lifestyles; ensure high quality health services that are efficient and accessible; integrate renewal of the health care system with longer term plans in the areas of prevention, health promotion and protection; reduce health inequalities in Canadian society; and provide health information to help Canadians make informed decisions."[2]

Unspoken Secret: The reason that Canada's health care spending increases are lower than other countries is that it plays hardball with its citizens.

Each provincial government administers health care within its borders, financed with tax money collected by the Canadian federal government. The federal government sets a global budget for each province, and the province is limited by that budget as to how much it can spend. A global budget is the total amount of money available to spend across the entire system for each fiscal year. In other words, the federal government tells each province how much money it will get to provide health care services each year – and no more. If the money runs out before the end of the budget period, so does the citizens' health care. This produces health care rationing – a direct result of how Health Canada controls spending.

Provincial government bureaucrats are the officials charged with operating the global budget. This makes the provincial health care administrator the government health care gatekeeper.

1. "About Health Care," *About Missions, Values,* Activities, http://www.hc-sc.gc/ahc-asc/activit/aboutapropros/index_e.html
2. Ibid.

If the provincial administrator fails to control spending, the Canadian federal government can withhold money from that province. So the provinces that might suffer greater sickness, or that fail to hold down costs, are further penalized by losing even more federal revenue. The irony is that it is the federal government that sets the global budget, and if it is set too low, it is the provincial citizens that will suffer from fewer health care services the following budget period.

Health Canada discovered years ago that it cannot afford every health care benefit that its citizens desire. Its primary method of controlling health care costs is to limit availability of services – rationing.

"Citizens of Canada, for example, have no right to any particular health care service. They have no right to an MRI scan. They have no right to heart surgery. They do not even have the right to a place in line. The 100th person waiting for heart surgery is not entitled to the 100th surgery. Other people can and do jump the queue. One could even argue that Canadians have fewer rights to health services than their pets. While Canadian pet owners can purchase an MRI scan for their cat or dog, purchasing a scan for themselves is illegal."[3]

In fact, it is illegal for Canadians to use their own money to purchase any health care services outside of what the government has approved. Why? To allow citizens to make private health care purchases defeats the fairness doctrine. It is unfair for one member of society to have more than another. Since not everyone else can afford additional health care services, no one should be allowed to do so. For one citizen to be free to have more than others is considered wrong and immoral. It is the ultimate violation of the fairness doctrine in a socialized, single-payer, health

---

3. John C. Goodman, *Health Care in a Free Society, Rebutting the Myths of National Health Insurance,* the National Center for Policy Analysis, Dallas, TX, Jan. 27, 2005, 2-3.

care system. To us, it is unimaginable that a government gatekeeper could prohibit parents from spending their own money to buy additional life-saving health care for their child. We would never tolerate this.

If Health Canada allowed people to purchase health services on their own, it would increase the pressure to move the system toward private health insurance; they are not yet quite ready to do so. Canada is still far too early in the evolutionary cycle which would move them from strict government control to some level of free market health care.

So what do Canadians do when they are denied care "back home?"

HOW WILL MARY GET HER NEW KNEE?

"Why can't I get an artificial knee like my cousin Sally in the United States?" Mary, the Canadian grandmother, asks.

"Well, we have determined this is not a need. You are not entitled to a new knee because you can still walk, and besides, we have already spent our annual budget for knee surgeries," the gatekeeper explains. "Unless you want to pay more taxes, you will have to wait. The country wants to keep its health care spending at less than 10 percent, you know."

"I have saved enough to pay it out of my own pocket," Mary says, rubbing her sore knee.

"Oh no, that is illegal. That would be unfair to others who cannot pay."

Mary flew to Detroit a month later, claiming that she was taking a vacation. While there, she purchased knee surgery. The knee that Mary wanted and the technique to install it were developed in the U.S. as a result of medical research, and it was widely available.

Unspoken Secret: Health Canada spends more than $1 billion a year on health care services purchased in the United States.[4] They do this because of a shortage of certain critical care facilities and physicians, such as heart surgeons and adequate cancer care. Beyond this $1 billion, it is unknown how much of their personal money private Canadian citizens spend in U.S. health facilities. By this, Health Canada admits that its system cannot adequately meet its people's needs, and it must turn to the U.S., where free markets have created more health care options.

WE'LL GET THAT TEST...SOON...WE HOPE

In Canada, there are severe shortages of diagnostic devices, often forcing patients to wait months for a test. "In total, the estimated 815,663 Canadians waiting for treatment in 2004 waited a combined 11.3 million weeks."[5] This calculates to more than three months of waiting for a test. Some Canadians become sicker while waiting, perhaps moving from serious to critical condition.

Waiting so long for care also means that some Canadians lose wages as they are forced to skip work at least some of the time. In 2004 this lost income cost "... $9,150 per patient for the estimated 9.8 percent of patients suffering considerable hardships while waiting."[6] This amounted to an average of $2,700 per person on the waiting lists.[7]

Even though they may have to wait, all Canadian citizens are entitled to see a doctor if they want to, but they get little time with their physician. Canadian doctors, whose

---

4. Ibid., 7.
5. Nadeem Esmail, "The Private Cost of Public Queues," Fraser Institute, March 2005, 28.
6. Ibid.
7. Ibid., 29.

numbers are artificially limited by the College of Physicians and Surgeons, see an average of 3,143 patients a year. U.S. doctors see 2,222. That means that Canadian doctors see 41 percent more patients than their U.S. counterparts.[8]

THESE MAY BE THE FIRST STEPS
AWAY FROM SOCIALIZED HEALTH CARE

It is illegal to buy private health insurance for hospital and physician charges in Canada. During 2005, however, the Canadian Supreme Court weighed in, ruling that Quebec's citizens do have a right to purchase private health insurance.

Quebec citizens apparently have come to question the fairness doctrine, concluding that they have the moral right to make more of their own health care decisions. They want to choose how to spend more of their own money on health care – they want personal choice, not more taxes or state control.

This court decision will spark a lively and divisive debate in the Canadian Parliament centered on the fairness doctrine. Is it now to be considered fair that people with more money will be allowed to purchase private insurance and gain access to more or better health care services? Or, will the Canadian socialists win the debate and overturn the court's decision? (In Canada, socialists are open about their economic ideology, and consistently win parliamentary seats. In America, to openly declare that you are a socialist will cost votes, except for Vermont's Bernard Sanders.)

A Vancouver medical clinic has, likewise, recently incurred the wrath of Canadian socialists. They are angry because the new clinic offers more and better health care services to people who are willing to purchase an annual

---

8. See note 3, 8.

membership. The clinic promises, in return, to provide high -quality, readily available services, even though provincial health care funds will pay the charges. The socialists are angry because they see that this clinic creates a two-tiered health system – one for the masses, and a second for those with higher income or more assets. The socialists believe this is unfair and immoral.

Canadians pay for their prescription drugs either without insurance, or with insurance that provides limited coverage and high deductibles. (See chapter 10 for a more complete explanation of the Canadian drug benefit plan.) The effect of the high dollars Canadians pay out-of-pocket is to force the drug companies to set their prices low. In the U.S., a good portion of the cost of prescription drugs is paid by the government or private insurance, so that Americans are shielded from the real cost of their medicines.

Though thousands of Canadians travel to the U.S. for critical health care services, there are good reasons that we do not read about U.S. residents going to Canada for health care. Our system provides far more, and timely diagnostic, surgical, and life-saving services.

Once they do get to see the doctor, Canadians enjoy a good quality of health care services, but must pay high federal taxes for this privilege – it is far from free. The system has a good reputation for preventive care, but fails for sick or critical care, especially that which demands diagnostic and surgical services.

Unspoken Secret: In a single-payer system such as in Canada, inevitably those who are quite ill and need the most care will suffer discrimination, only it will come in the form of being denied life-saving health care. This is the greatest failing of the fairness doctrine, leaving the most vulnerable patients without the services they would purchase on their own, if the government allowed it.

Americans who believe that the Canadian system would be an improvement over our system because of their belief in the fairness doctrine, need to understand that they would be denying health care services to those who need them the most. That rubs most of us as wrong. In the United States, our free market system responds to everyone who needs health care – we believe in access to health care, and especially for sick people.

Next, we examine the United Kingdom's system, one that spends the least per capita and the lowest of the five as a fraction of GDP (half of the U.S.). It is a more mature socialist system than is Canada. How have they managed to keep spending so low?

CHAPTER 16
UNITED KINGDOM
(BRITISH) HEALTH CARE

The United Kingdom's 60 million citizens live in a country of 145,900 square miles, slightly smaller than California (California's population is about 36 million). The UK spends $137 billion, 7.7 percent of its $1.78 trillion GDP on health care, spending less of their GDP on health care than do the other five countries we studied.

World War II left UK neighborhoods devastated from German bombs. Hundreds of thousands of her soldiers lay dead on battlefields across Europe. Other soldiers bore the scars of war, and returned home to a country in shambles and a medical system under extreme stress.

At the same time, UK citizens witnessed a parade of new medical discoveries. This created demand for new, expensive therapies and surgeries. "More mothers were wanting their babies delivered in hospitals, cardiac surgery was being applied to rheumatic heart disease, and the first hip replacements were beginning to be performed."[1]

As a result, UK lawmakers created a free, socialized public health care system in 1948 – the National Health

---

1. http://www.nhs.uk/England/AboutThe Nhs/History/1948-1957.cmsx

Service (NHS). The lawmakers granted the NHS monopoly control over the nation's health. They meant to let the NHS be the UK's single payer. Everyone would receive the same care at no personal cost. In many ways, this reflects how the Canadian system looked at its beginning.

As the UK system matured during the next 55-plus years, it found that it could not rely strictly on socialized medicine. We will show you how.

COST EFFECTIVE HEALTH CARE

"It is difficult today for us to imagine," says the NHS, "what life must have been like without free health care and the difference that the arrival of the NHS made to people's lives."[2] This imagination suffers from reality.

"Many of the tensions that emerged in the early days of the NHS have challenged its senior management and successive governments ever since." The challenges are "...how to fund it adequately, how to balance the often conflicting demands and expectations of patients, staff and taxpayers, how to ensure finite resources are targeted where they are most needed..."[3]

The authors thank the British for being so open and honest about their system. In this quote, we see that from its beginning, NHS managers had to define what it meant to offer cost-effective health care. Cost-effective health care means trying to find a way to meet the people's needs with limited, even severely limited, financial resources. It means planning which services to offer, which to ignore, and at its worst, allowing some people to die, or not allowing others to be born (see chapter 11). Cost-effective health care puts the system first, not the people's needs.

---

2. http://www.nhs.uk/England/AboutThe Nhs/History/Before1948.cmsx
3. See note 1, "Balancing Demands."

The two least cost-effective treatments might be delivering and treating a premature baby, or providing for those suffering from cancer. Government gatekeepers know that the best return on their dollars is providing preventive care. Preventive care is low-cost, and hopefully, provides long-term health. (To the NHS manager, it means saving money in the future.)

Children receive the highest volume of preventive health services. This comes in the form of prenatal and pediatric care. It also includes a battery of vaccinations designed to keep those little people from getting sick, both early and later in life. Vaccinations, then, are cost-effective.

The authors are most concerned in this book about everyone receiving high-quality health care when they need it. We do not subscribe to the idea of providing health care based on a strict, cost-effective analysis. That said, however, government-controlled health care systems do evaluate services based on cost, and by doing so, limit services provided to their populations. The authors do not want this to become the norm in the United States. We show in the following paragraphs just how dangerous it is.

As we showed earlier, the cost of caring for one premature baby, that can run to $750,000 or more, could purchase an entire vaccination set for 1,875 children. The cost of a full battery of vaccinations spread over a child's lifetime averages out to about $5.15 a year.[4] The government gatekeeper analyzing this from a strict cost effective standpoint may decide it is better that those premature babies not be allowed to be born, so that nearly 2,000 children can be vaccinated.

Compared to the relatively inexpensive cost of preventive care for infants and toddlers, we ask what might be the least cost-effective health care service? Perhaps it would be

---

4. $400 total cost of vaccinations spread over the current life expectancy of 77.6 years.

for the 90-year old grandmother who needs a new hip at a cost of $40,000 or more.[5] The gatekeeper denies her that care, however, because she likely will die in a few years. The new hip is not cost effective.

In the middle of the two extremes – preventive care for children and a new hip for an aging grandmother – lies cancer. Cancer is most certainly the least cost effective of all diseases. It takes enormous revenues to treat a cancer victim, and in many cases the person will die prematurely. Providing cancer care is, then, not cost effective. There is little reason to wonder that "...25,000 people die unnecessarily in Britain each year because they are denied the highest quality cancer care."[6]

They are denied cancer care for two reasons. First, there are long waiting times between early suspicion of the cancer and the onset of treatment. The NHS' goal is for all patients diagnosed with cancer to begin treatments by two months after it is first suspected.[7] This goal is a broad average, meaning that some patients will wait far longer. Also, this is a most recent goal, a result of the UK's poor performance for cancer victims in the past.

Secondly, the patient whose general practice doctor first discovers the cancer faces another obstacle: the UK has a severe shortage of oncologists, "...fewer oncologists than any country in Western Europe."[8] The government is the agency that determines how many oncologists will be trained, and the NHS has tried to control health care spending by limiting the supply of doctors; hence, the shortage of oncologists.

<u>Unspoken Secret</u>: U.S. advocates of single-payer

---

5. Medica Insurance Company underwriter, 12/15/2005, via telephone. Allina Health Care Systems, 12/15/2005, via telephone.
6. John C. Goodman, "Health Care in a Free Society, Rebutting the Myths of National Health Insurance," National Center for Policy Analysis, Dallas, TX, Jan. 27, 2005," 6.
7. "Performance Indicators for Acute and Specialist Trust," http://nhs.uk/England/About-TheNhs/StarRatings/AcuteSpecialPI.cmsx, 4.
8. See note 6, 8.

health care that would resemble the United Kingdom's system, often claim that 18,000 uninsured Americans die prematurely because they lack health insurance – 18,000 out of a population of 294 million. That compares with 25,000 British, out of a population of 60 million that die from cancer, because the NHS-controlled system has a shortage of cancer doctors. If that same cancer death ratio applied to the U.S., it would mean 122,000 people dying from cancer *just because there are not enough oncologists* – and that does not happen.

Let's stop and look toward home for a minute. When we consider how to spend our own money, we have to count the cost of everything. That means eliminating some activities, putting off buying a new car, or, perhaps staying in a smaller home. Our money only stretches so far.

Cost-effective health care is like a family budget. Anything considered to be less than cost effective must be eliminated: cancer victims will be denied life-preserving care because it is not cost effective. When we talk about human life, though, where do we draw the line? If the National Health Service has limited money available, is it more cost effective to spend it on treatment for chronic asthma, or for a person with aggressive liver cancer?

Yes, the UK spends half of what we do in the U.S. It has determined that health care resources are limited. In the United States, we have not set such a limit. We will take care of that premature baby, provide vaccinations, help the asthma sufferer, give grandma her hip, and do everything we can for cancer victims. We spend what it takes, not what the government has predetermined.

FAIR, FREE CARE GOT TO BE EXPENSIVE

Only a short time passed before the UK's free health care system found itself falling short of cash to pay the mounting bills. "Within three years of its creation, the NHS was forced to introduce some modest fees. Prescription charges of one shilling...were introduced in 1952. A flat rate of £1 [one pound] for ordinary dental treatment was brought in at the same time."[9]

As the demand for NHS services grew, so did its administrative costs. The Service is operated under guidelines set by a National Health Board that currently has 1.3 million employees,[10] and is the largest employer in the UK. The family practice doctor is the NHS gatekeeper, controlling access to all other health care services. UK doctors treat far more patients a year than U.S doctors – an average of 3,176 per year as compared to 2,222 in the U.S.,[11] meaning that they see 43 percent more patients than U.S. doctors, even more than Canadian doctors. The UK's free care encourages this increased utilization, but robs the system of money it needs for critical care. "More than one million people are waiting for medical treatment in UK hospitals at any one time, and an estimated 500,000 surgeries were cancelled in the past five years because of the shortage of NHS hospital beds."[12]

During the late 1960s and into the 1980s, the NHS faced increasing pressure from the same forces as did the U.S. health care system. Medical breakthroughs in technology, surgery, and pharmaceuticals sent demand and costs soaring. Unlike America, where the free market allowed capitalists and a huge middle class to invest hundreds of billions of dollars in innovation, new private insurance models, and new health care strategies, the NHS looked to the central government for solutions. To maintain its sense of fairness, while not allowing wealthier people to pur-

9. See note 1.
10. "Leading expert calls for NHS to tackle soaring levels of workforce stress," June 17, 2005, http://www.nhsconfed.org/press/releases/workforce_stress.asp
11. See note 6, 4.
12. Ibid., 12.

chase private insurance, the government had four options: reduce benefits, reduce the number of health care providers, increase taxes, or create health care system efficiencies designed to reduce cost.[13]

The NHS hoped that these late 1970s reforms would slow the upward spiraling of health care costs by showing which medical providers were efficient. The NHS refused to address the real issue; the idea that health care was free, and people used it too frequently. Since they clung to their refusal to allow anyone to spend their own money on additional health care services, they could only turn to health care rationing. The NHS single-payer system had sprung financial leaks that threatened to drown it in a sea of red ink, or penalize sick people to reduce and control costs.

Just 40 years after they created it, by the late 1980s, UK politicians had found that their health care system was beset by debt. Waiting lists for necessary services had grown, and they had to close down debt-ridden hospitals. The fairness doctrine had to change or the system would go broke.

FINALLY, A LITTLE FREE MARKET LIGHT BROKE THROUGH

The debate over the fairness doctrine raged, and the free market finally won an important battle. This is similar to the current debate in Canada.

The politicians voted to allow a limited free market system in which physicians were allowed to offer private health care. This meant that people with discretionary income would be allowed to spend their money on their own health care. Prior to this law change, UK residents were not allowed to purchase private health care services –

---

13. http://www.nhs.uk?England/AboutTheNhs/History/1978-1987.cmsx.

to do so violated the fairness doctrine, because some people might get more or better health care than others.

Under this new plan, doctors could purchase services from the government-owned facilities and suppliers, but sell their services to privately funded patients. This created a private health insurance market, and attracted badly needed capital into the health care system. As a result, today 13 percent of UK residents own private insurance.[14]

This created competition within the system. Those doctors who were better business operators provided higher quality services to their patients, creating a two-tiered health care system. Now with private insurance, the system had to respond to the needs of those 13 percent who owned it, rather than to just follow the cost-effective guidelines of the state system. The providers now had freedom to work with the patient to develop a plan of care, because the patient's insurance paid their bills, not the NHS.

TWO TIERS: GOVERNMENT-PAID OR NON-GOVERNMENT-PAID

Eighty-seven percent of British people continued to receive health care paid for by the NHS, while 13 percent had it from private insurance. The 87 percent received tier one care, typified by rationing and waiting lines. The 13 percent received tier two care, more like what we in the U.S. enjoy, without waiting lines, and actually receiving the promised benefits.

It only took a short time for the 87 percent to envy the better benefits available to the 13 percent. This created competition unfamiliar to the NHS monopoly. Competition forced the NHS to actually attempt to deliver the care that it had long promised, or pretended, to offer. People saw the

14. See note 6, 6-7.

difference between what they received and what the 13 percent received – and wanted it.

During the 1990s, spending increased dramatically as the NHS tried to deliver more health services to satisfy its enrollees.

As is the nature of government agencies, the NHS formed the National Service Frameworks (NSF) to study the system and recommend reforms. The NSF recommended upgrading data collection information and putting patients' medical records online for access by their doctors. They pledged to hire more medical staff, provide cleaner hospitals, and serve better food. Most notably, they did not recommend further privatization of UK health care. They wanted to retain the government monopoly.

The NSF felt proud that it could offer choices to NHS patients. "From the summer 2004 patients who will wait more than six months for elective surgery will be offered the choice of moving to another hospital for faster treatment."[15]

In the UK, health care choice means going to a different medical provider if the first one fails to schedule the patient for more than six months. By the time the patient finds a willing hospital with an opening, it could be too late. Small irritations can grow into deadly diseases.

In 2003, the NHS created a rating system to evaluate medical providers. They named it "Star Ratings." The Star Ratings provide several benchmarks that providers are to strive to attain. Clearly, the UK is fighting to retain its fairness doctrine for the 87 percent still locked into the NHS, government-gatekeeper system. It is hoped that this will allow the country to hold down overall health care spending.

---

15. "Choice for patients who have waited six months," http://www.dh.uk/PolicyAndGuid-ance/PatientChoice/Choice/ChoiceArticle/fs/en?CONTENT_ID=4065544&chk=Puc11A.

So In the UK You Get What You Pay For

High tech equipment is available to UK patients, but not as it is in the U.S. The NHS owns about half as many MRI units and CT scanners per million patients as do U.S. health care providers.[16] The UK has determined that it is not cost effective to have a surplus of these machines, but lack of a surplus also means that many UK patients are denied the timely use of the best diagnostic equipment. Such delays can mean the difference between life and death, or needlessly extending pain and suffering.

Affordability and access are touted as benefits of this government-controlled system, yet the government has realized it takes the availability of private health insurance to meet citizens' needs. Single-payer health care advocates praise the United Kingdom's low level of spending, ignoring the severe and serious shortages in critical care medicine it has created.

Americans will not tolerate these critical shortages, and it is one of the reasons we spend more on health care than they do. We understand that we will get the kind of care for which we pay. Our strong economy makes this possible, but if our economy ever falters or collapses, or if our cities are devastated by war, we, too, might demand that the government take over health care.

---

16. See note 6, 5-6.

CHAPTER 17
LAND OF LONG LIVES: JAPANESE HEALTH CARE

Japan's 127 million citizens live in a country of 145,900 square miles, the same land mass as the United Kingdom and slightly smaller than California. The Japanese spend $366 billion, 7.9 percent of their $3.7 trillion GDP on health care. Why is it that the Japanese spend half as much per capita as is spent in the U.S., and yet they enjoy the longest life expectancy in the world?

The Japanese health care system might seem to many of us to be caught in a time warp. In many ways it resembles the U.S. health care system of 50 years ago, in how it pays its bills. "Japan has an advantage over many other health systems because it...imposes relatively high levels of co-payments."[1] The Japanese face co-insurance cost of as much as 30 percent, and pay an average of 44 percent of the cost of employer-based health insurance premiums.

Many insured benefits we take for granted are not covered under the Japanese system. "In Japan, pregnancy is viewed as a voluntary condition," so childbirth expenses

---

1. Peter C. Smith, "Health care reforms in Europe and their implications for Japan," *The Japanese Journal of Social Security Policy: Vol. 3, No. 2,* Dec. 2004, 93.

are not covered by insurance.[2] Neither are "[h]ealth exams and check-ups...,"[3] or prosthetics.[4] And the Japanese pay for their own vaccinations. The U.S. health care system, likewise, did not cover these services until the early 1980s.

Like our earliest Americans, the Japanese still believe strongly in the work ethic and in close-knit, supportive families. That may account for the near-microscopic number of people for whom the government purchases health insurance. "...[T]he central government, together with local governments, provides the Medical Aid program for the very poor who would otherwise have difficulty in affording their co-payments...The number of Medical Aid recipients was 0.8 million in 1999, 0.6% of the whole population..."[5] Just over 1 million Japanese participate in Public Assistance programs. (In the U.S., various government units pay for the health care of more than 36.5 million non-Medicare recipients, 12.4 percent of the population.)

The Japanese family "...stretching back three generations..."[6] can receive health benefits from one, consolidated health insurance policy. Those who qualify must receive the majority of their support from the breadwinner. The Japanese idea that such large family groups should be covered under the same policy is remarkable, given how western nations have gone in the other direction, with family members almost always living independently of each other.

The Japanese system has no global budget. The system will spend whatever it takes to care for its people. Without such a restraint, the Japanese are the world's leader in providing treatment for kidney failure. Their combined dialsis

2. Tomoko Furukawa, "Health Care Puzzles," *The Japan Times Online*, Nov. 16, 2004.
3. Tomoko Furukawa, "A Primer on Health Care," *The Japan Times Online*, Nov. 9, 2004.
4. "Healthcare System," Japan Pharmaceutical Manufacturers Association, http://www.jpma.or.jp/12english/guide_industry/healthcare/healthcare.html.
5. "Labour Market and Social Policy, Occasional Papers No 56: An Assessment of the Performance of the Japanese Health Care System," Directorate for Education, Employment, Labour, and Social Affairs Committee, OECD, Dec. 2001, para 34, 20-21.
6. See note 3.

and transplant rate is one-third greater than in the U.S. (the second leading provider of these services) and three times that of the world's average.[7] By this, the Japanese show that they invest in people, and in part, it helps explain their longer life expectancy.

Japan leads the world in life expectancy at 81.8 years.[8] It has an infant mortality rate of just 3.3 deaths per 1,000 live births,[9] even though neither prenatal, childbirth, postnatal, nor postpartum care are covered by health insurance. At least in Japan, this contradicts the argument that pregnant women without health insurance will suffer higher infant mortality. There must be other factors at work; we believe it is directly related to their culture and genetics.

With all of Japan's successes, however, American advocates of a single-payer government-run system seldom mention Japanese health care as an ideal model. It relies far too much on out-of-pocket payments, free markets, free will, fee-for-service, and private insurance for the comfort of those who prefer a government-run health care system.

In chapter 12 we discussed how Japanese heredity and culture affect health, especially life expectancy. A great deal of their success, both in terms of long lives and relatively good health, accrues as much to genetics and culture as it does to the effectiveness of their health care system.

FUNDING THE JAPANESE HEALTH CARE SYSTEM

Every Japanese resident is expected to own health insurance, and their uninsured rate is nearly non-existent. A large majority receive their health insurance through a gov-

---

7. See note 5, Table 14, 50.
8. OECD Life Expectancy Tables, June 2005.
9. "Infant Mortality and Life Expectancy for Selected Countries, 2004," U.S. Census Bureau, International Data Base, infoplease.com.

ernment program, although most pay insurance premiums to one of the countries 5,000 private insurance companies.

The Japanese system is funded by insurance premiums, taxes, and significant out-of-pocket expenses. Employed persons pay, on the average, 44 percent of the premium cost of their health insurance, with the employers paying the remaining 56 percent.[10] The annual disposable income of an employed Japanese worker averages $17,267 compared to $27,142 in the U.S.[11] Though the government caps the total premium a person could pay each year, the maximum amount can be as much as 530,000 yen (even more for wealthier citizens), or about US$4,560.[12] That is the same as an American paying $7,168 per year for insurance premiums.

When the Japanese use health care services, insurance covers 70 percent of their bill (depending on the type of insurance they own), and the employee pays the 30 percent not covered by insurance. These co-insurance costs are capped at 63,000 yen per month – about $542. There is a formula for long-term expenses during a calendar year that limits total out-of-pocket payments to about US$4,500.[13]

So the maximum financial exposure for a typical middle-class Japanese worker in a year is capped at about US$9,060. This would be the same as an American worker paying $14,241 in a year. So, if America copied the Japanese health insurance system, it would expose the average U.S. income earner to a potential health cost exceeding 50 percent of their annual disposable income.

Japan has learned that to control health care spending, each citizen must bear a good portion of the potential cost, instead of being entitled to having 100 percent of health costs paid by someone else.

10. See note 5, 15.
11. For 2003, "Basic Structural Statistics," Main Economic Indicators, 2005, OECD, 1.
12. See note 3.
13. Ibid.

Because they have a great potential exposure to costs, Japanese "[p]atients have a degree of financial incentive to economize since they make co-payments, as determined by the health insurance Fee Schedule...,"[14] and the fee schedule must be kept low so that citizens can afford their co-payments. These factors may be the key to Japan's ability to hold down national health care spending. In the U.S., where co-payments are low, health care consumers have very little incentive to hold down spending. This makes health care appear to be free or almost free, and provides no sense of spending restraint as in Japan.

The Japanese citizen knows what their costs are for health care services. Combined with their culture, ethnicity and genetics, paying a good portion of their own bills provides a financial incentive to take better care of themselves and their families.

NATIONAL HEALTH CARE DATES TO 1927

Japan's first form of national health insurance dates to 1927, though it only covered employers with 10 or more employees. By 1961, Japan had made health insurance mandatory for everyone. To ease the financial burden, the government placed a cap on the dollar amount any citizen would pay for care each year, as described above.

The Japanese have had a senior health care insurance program similar to Medicare since the 1970s, but in Japan, one must be at least 70 to enroll. The plan requires a significant premium payment, and co-insurance costs, as a means to hold down overall spending.

"With a rapidly aging population, reforms in recent years have focused on improving access to health and long

---

14. See note 5, 15.

term care services by the elderly and on shifting the balance of long term care away from hospitals towards nursing homes and domiciliary settings."[15] Traditionally, Japanese seniors have lived out their final days in hospitals, not nursing homes. Continuing cost pressure during the 1990s has forced the Japanese government to create Long Term Health Care Insurance – they wanted to move away from hospital facilities to nursing homes, as they demanded that seniors pay for more of the cost of their own health care.

Japanese officials recently began requiring seniors to pay for 10 percent of their personal health care costs. This is to offset increased taxes and premiums paid by workers, a burden that has made it more difficult for Japanese businesses to compete worldwide, and for families to care for their own needs.

JAPANESE HEALTH CARE FACTS AND FIGURES

The Japanese system does not rely on a single payer. Health insurance is sold by more than 5,000 private insurance companies, and those companies pay a large share of the nation's health care bills.

The national government determines which benefits will be offered and sets the prices. This means there is no difference in which services are covered and not covered by Japan's insurers. Premium cost differences between insurance companies will vary somewhat, as the Japanese system of competition between insurance companies applies pressure to hold down insurance costs.

The national government leaves many decisions to local authorities, including the number of hospital beds

---

15. Ibid., 4.

available in cities and towns.[16] This allows the system to be more democratic in that local authorities have the knowledge, understanding, and close contact required to make good decisions on behalf of their citizens.

The selling price of health care services is set by a government committee comprised of doctors, patients' representatives, insurance companies, and government officials.

Japanese people see their doctor more often than in any other country other than in Hungary: an average of nearly 16 times a year. Americans average 5.8 visits per year.[17] In fact, a Japanese doctor conducts nearly 8,900 consultations a year, compared with 2,222 for American doctors. Doctors bill insurance companies for each visit, so to make up for the low fee allowed per visit, they see patients more often. This large number of patient visits to the doctor also may be attributed to the fact that Japanese physicians supply most of the country's prescription drugs. This allows the doctor to more closely monitor patient outcomes, positive or negative, and make adjustments in medications as needs arise.

The doctor is readily available, and sees patients whether or not they have appointments. "…[T]he Japanese do not wait for health services (Esmail and Walker, 2004, A. Joeng and Hurst, 2001). The health care services that Japanese citizens require are readily available with virtually no waiting time."[18]

We saw that Canada, with its single-payer system, holds health care spending at about 10 percent of GDP. At the same time, Japan sat at about eight percent of its GDP (although the Japanese spending rate has grown rapidly during the past 10 years). Japan, relying on private insurance and high out-of-pocket costs, does not suffer the long

16. Ibid., 21.
17. Ibid., 40.
18. Nadeem Esmail, "Look to Japan on Health," Fraser Forum, Nov. 2004.

waiting lines common to Canada. Japan, as well, has an abundance of CT scanners, more than 10 times that of Canada, per capita.[19]

The Japanese government controls the number and type of physicians admitted to its government medical schools, but private medical schools are market driven, controlling their own admissions. Japanese physicians typically learn through a mentoring program, under the tutelage of experienced primary care doctors.

DOCTORS AND HOSPITALS

Private doctors work as for-profit businesses while most hospitals are non-profit entities. Hospitals employ their own doctors, so that unlike in the U.S., a person's private physician is usually not allowed to treat them in a hospital. As many as 30 percent of doctors have set up hospital beds in their own clinics, satisfying a need in the way that free markets adapt.

Hospitalized patients must pay directly for their own food; they reason that they have to buy it at home, so why not in the hospital.

Once Japanese patients enter the hospital, they stay an average of 30.8 days,[20] compared to the U.S. where the average stay is 4.8 days.[21] Japan's length of stay is nearly three times that of the second-ranked nation, Switzerland. The average hospitalization data for Japan are distorted because of their cultural preference for seniors to spend their final days of life in the hospital. Seniors have been able to do this in the past because of low, to no, co-payments. To reduce length of hospital stays, the government is now requiring seniors to pay co-payments, making them

19. Ibid.
20. See note 5, 41.
21. "Average Length of Stay by Diagnostic Category, 2003, QuickStats," U.S. Centers for Disease Control, http://www.cdc.gov/mmwr?preview/mmwrhtml/mm5427a6.htm

more aware of the costs of treatment, and encouraging them to move to long term care facilities. Just like people everywhere, when the service appeared to be free, Japanese seniors took advantage of it.

Japanese hospitals are more crowded than are U.S. hospitals, with only about one-third the floor space per bed. Japanese citizens are free to choose any doctor they wish, but they are not like U.S. primary care doctors who often refer patients to specialists. Japanese doctors treat everything; there are very few specialists.

HIGH PRESCRIPTION DRUG USE

"Moreover, doctors can both prescribe and dispense drugs..."[22] and they do so, quite liberally.

Japan ranks among the highest in the world for expenditures on drugs as a percentage of its total health care spending – 18.4 percent, compared to 12.9 percent in America.[23] However, on a per person basis, the Japanese spend US$530, but in the U.S., spending is about $180 more, at $710 per person.[24]

The government has been trying to wean patients off buying drugs from their doctors, by squeezing profit margins and raising co-insurance. The most important reason, however, that Japanese pharmaceutical costs are soaring is not the cost of drugs, but the escalating level of drug consumption – more people using more drugs, just as in the United States.

---

22. See note 5, para 19, 15.
23. "Health Spending and Resources," OECD in Figures, 2005 edition.
http://oecd.p4.siteinterent.com/publications/doifiles/012005061T002.xls.
24. 18.4% of $366 billion, divided by 127 million population, compared to 12.9% of $1.7 trillion, divided by 296 million population (numbers are rounded).

SO WHY NOT LOOK TO THE JAPANESE?

If the purpose of health care reform is to reduce health care spending, then it might be expected that reformers would look to Japan for answers. They do not. Here is why:

    1. Japanese culture demands personal responsibility and believes that all able-bodied persons should work. The Japanese enjoy the world's longest life expectancy, low infant mortality, and almost zero uninsured. The Japanese culture frowns on public welfare programs, so that the government pays co-payments for less than one percent of the population.

    2. Individuals take personal responsibility for a great deal of their own health care costs, paid through co-payments and co-insurance. Many health care services must be paid out of pocket, even childbirth and vaccinations. Extended families continue to support each other, and that includes providing health insurance reaching back three generations.

    3. Competition is encouraged. Japan has 5,000 private insurance companies, doctors are for-profit and compete with each other for business. They are paid on a fee-for-service basis. Local governments make decisions about the supply of hospital beds. There are no government-imposed global budgets, and no gatekeeper doctors. Private medical schools control their own admissions, and new doctors are mentored by more experienced doctors.

The reason liberal U.S. reformers ignore the Japanese system is because it relies so much on market forces. The Japanese citizen pays a significant part of his or her own bills out of pocket, that could amount to as much as half their income in an unhealthy year. The Japanese citizen knows what health care costs.

The idea that individuals should pay a large portion of their own health costs out of pocket has very little appeal to liberal U.S. health care reformers. They prefer to blame insurance companies, doctors, hospitals, or Big Pharma, rather than to face the fact that the entitlement mentality, driven by the fairness doctrine, is the chief problem of U.S. health care spending. In Japan, everyone is entitled and expected to find a job, take care of their families, and pay their own bills.

CHAPTER 18
WORLD'S BEST SYSTEM: FRENCH HEALTH CARE
INTERNATIONAL POLITICS TRIES
TO INFLUENCE HEALTH CARE SYSTEMS

France's 60 million citizens live in a country of 211,200 square miles, 30,000 square miles smaller than Texas. The French spend $174 billion, 10.1 percent of their $1.72 trillion GDP on health care.

During 2000, the World Health Organization (WHO) "...ranked the French health care system number one among the 191 member countries surveyed..."[1] The World Health Organization is "the United Nations specialized agency for health."[2] As an organization, the U.N. has long favored socialist countries, and often holds the United States in contempt.

The WHO ranking took into consideration five criteria:

    1. "...overall level of health within a population;

    2. health inequalities within a population [how much economic status affects health];

---

1. Patrick Lenain, "Santé to the French health system," Economics department, October 2000, http://www.oecdobserver.org/news/fullstory.php/aid/356/ Sant%E9_to_the_French_health_system_.html.
2. About WHO, http://www.who.int/about/en/

　　3.　health system responsiveness [patient satisfaction];

　　4.　responsiveness within the population [how well people in various economic groups are served]; and

　　5.　distribution of costs [who pays the bills]."[3]

The same 2000 WHO survey listed U.S. health care at number 37. The WHO placed great significance on its subjective judgment of what a fair view of distribution of health care services looks like (it prefers that everyone should receive the same services on the same basis).

Concern for the poor caught the French politicians' ears in 2000, as the French Parliament mandated a form of publicly financed health insurance for 10 percent of their residents. Unlike those who have to make co-payments, France's poorest residents enjoy 100 percent coverage, and doctors are locked into charging them prices set by the government. This resembles the U.S. Medicaid system.

"The plan therefore provides health care to those that were previously deprived or badly insured, including persons in unstable employment situations, or foreigners waiting for official residency papers."[4] The French, like the Canadians, and unlike in the U.S., refuse to pay the health care costs of illegal immigrants.

As they rate countries, the WHO also places great weight on infant mortality and life expectancy statistics, ignoring critical issues such as dietary habits, genetics, and culture. It ignores the fact that the U.S. birth rate is higher and death rate lower than that of the French, and these two facts speak volumes about our drive to preserve the tiniest

---

3. See note 1.
4. Ibid.

2004 Birth and Death Rates
Selected Countries[5]

Country	Birth Rate (per 1,000)	Death Rate (per 1,000)
United States	14.1	8.3
France	12.3	9.1
Germany	8.4	10.4
United Kingdom	10.9	10.2
Japan	9.6	8.8
Czech Republic	9.1	10.5

and sickest persons among us.

Since 2000, things have deteriorated in France. A 2004 WHO bulletin reported that "[p]roblems with the French public health care system became increasingly apparent in recent months. When Europe sweltered under a heat wave last August, for example, more than 15,000 people died in France, dwarfing the number of deaths in neighboring countries."[6] It is hard to imagine that the WHO failed to cry out against this terrible loss, but to do so would have meant condemning a government-controlled system. If the U.S. health care system produces a handful of persons who die due to the failure of a drug or a medical device, or after a Category 5 hurricane like Katrina, the entire world knows about it.

The centrist, socialized French health system is spared WHO scrutiny because it meets their view of what the ideal system should resemble. The U.S. health system, far more market-based, is always subjected to WHO suspicion and poor ratings, but who rates the World Health Organization? From its lofty 2000 accolades for the French system, the WHO gurus had to eat their hats during the next few years

---

5. "Crude Birth and Death Rates for Selected Countries," (per 1,000 population), infoplease.com
6. "Bulletin of the World Health Organization," March 2004, 232.

as, once again, socialized medicine failed to satisfy the citizens' needs.

BENEFITS INNER WORKINGS OF THE SYSTEMS

French legal residents receive health insurance through the country's social security system, and "...75% of total health spending is publicly funded."[7] Taxes are assessed against employers and employees (as are America's Social Security and Medicare taxes), plus individual income taxes pay an increasing share of the costs.

The ever-increasing share of the burden paid by income taxes is the result of an overall decrease in wage income. As France's economy falters and income drops, employers pay less into the system thereby robbing the national health insurance program of monies it needs to pay its bills. To make up for this lost revenue, France has been forced to resort to raising personal income taxes.[8] The government has also imposed price controls attempting to keep the system in balance, as it tries to make sure everyone gets their fair share of services.

Health insurance is provided mostly by private insurance companies, and these are managed jointly by employer groups and unions. The state referees between these powerful interests.

Health care funding is determined by the French parliament, but "...the cabinet decides reimbursement rates and sets the amount of contribution earmarked for the funds..."[9] French citizens have grown used to their socialist economy and seem comfortable with this concept.

Once politicians have established the global budget,

---

7. See note 1.
8. "The French Health Care System: A Brief Overview," Presentation prepared for the Permanent Working Group of European Junior Doctors, October 2001, 1.
9. Ibid.

then fund managers "...negotiate with health care professions to set tariffs [prices] designed to ensure the system operates at the breakeven point."[10] Since funds are predetermined and prices set in advance, the system responds poorly to unplanned events – such as deadly heat waves.

PRIVATE INSURANCE IS COMMON

About 85 percent of French residents purchase a supplemental insurance policy in the private market. Along with their co-payments, this covers the balance of their costs not paid by public health insurance.

The French system covers a broad range of services, even including "...stays in thermal spas."[11] These generous benefits have further caused costs to spiral upward. In an attempt to control them, the government increased co-payments to as much as 30-40 percent of the cost of care. "This tended to deter the poorest citizens...from seeking care,"[12] and that violates the French fairness doctrine whereby all residents are entitled to receive all the same services.

Doctors, trying to make up for lost revenue, also responded to those higher co-payments by increasing the number of services for which they billed. This reflects the problems associated with combining price fixing with the fairness doctrine; everyone must get the same services, but at artificially low prices set by the government.

French patients have free rein to choose any doctor they wish and go as often as they like. Health authorities are trying to put a stop to this practice by "... screening access to certain specialists and monitoring for flagrant over use."[13] Their limited resources drove them to put in

---

10. Ibid.
11. Ibid., 2.
12. Ibid.
13. See note 1, 2.

place a strict medical gatekeeper to hold down costs.

Yet, "flagrant over use" has grown into a crisis. The French High Council for the Future of Health Insurance issued a 2004 report where it identified "...a projected €10.9 billion (US $13.7 billion) shortfall in the public health insurance budget in 2004, which could balloon to nearly €66 billion (US $82.9 billion) by 2020."[14] In some ways, these projections parallel those of America's Medicare system, projected to run massive shortfalls at about the same time. Unlike the Canadians, the French continue to offer health services after exceeding the budget, and are willing to run a deficit to make sure that needs are met.

Price fixing has not solved the French deficit problem. They see what we enjoy in the U.S., and they want the same services. Since someone else pays most of their bills (government and supplemental insurance), they use a lot of services. The government's dilemma is that it cannot raise taxes any higher to fund all the "free" services demanded by their citizens.

The High Council also had to admit that the country's "system of refunding medical expenditures 'probably promotes some of the problems.' As a result, the French are bracing themselves for changes that will likely curb their liberal access to medical specialists, treatments and drugs. They will probably have to pay more, too."[15] Once again, the fairness doctrine of socialist health care systems may be forced to give way to human nature; people will use more of what they perceive to be free, and only by engaging them in the purchase of services will overall costs be reduced.

According to the 2004 WHO bulletin, the French system is rife with "[c]ompartmentalization, 'confusion about

14. See note 6.
15. Ibid.

who is in charge of what,' and a 'sometimes ridiculous accumulation of administration'..."[16] To further reduce costs, the French must reduce government administrative expenses, a very difficult task in any established public bureaucracy.

Hospitals are the core of the French system, placing emphasis on procedures to cure disease rather than prevent them. About 65 percent of hospital beds are owned by the government. "Private for-profit hospitals concentrate on surgical procedures and rely mostly on fee-for-service remuneration for their funding."[17] Eventually, all hospitals will be forced to conform to the same pricing structure whereby all aspects of a procedure will be pre-designated and paid for at a set price (called Diagnoses Related Guidelines – DRGs). DRGs have been used for decades in the U.S. for hospital pricing and billing.

French authorities have begun public campaigns to reduce drug and alcohol abuse and encourage healthier lifestyles.

Some French health care reformers want the government to fund 100 percent of an essential benefits set – services defined by the government as essential to everyone's basic health needs. This idea parallels what some American doctor groups are promoting. The essential benefits set idea meets the demands of the fairness doctrine; everyone getting the same care. The French, though, allow wealthier citizens to pay for anything else they want to purchase, even though such an idea violates the fairness doctrine.

DOCTORS' UNIONS FRUSTRATE HEALTH CARE OFFICIALS – REFORMS BEING IMPOSED FROM ABOVE

The French government sets the number of new doc-

16. Ibid.
17. See note 8.

tors allowed to be trained and retained, and most doctors belong to unions. The number of authorized doctors has been in recent decline, as the government tries to limit the supply of physicians to control costs.

Many French physicians prefer working in private practice where they are paid on a fee-for-service basis. This allows them more flexibility and independence than government-controlled doctors, but they still have little control over their fees which are "...set by experts and the prices are negotiated by physicians' unions and public health insurance funds."[18]

It took 26 years after the onset of the French public health care system for the doctors' unions to sign a contract with the government – in 1971. Their contracts are renegotiated every five years, but not without great rancor.

French doctors are bracing for a major overhaul of their system, called "Hospital 2007." Not all doctors are pleased, and since its 2004 inception, some doctors have gone on strike or orchestrated work slowdowns. It is impossible to conceive Americans tolerating a work slowdown forced upon our health care system by a doctor's union.

The WHO still praises the French system, but "[t]he realities of a rising financial burden and an aging population loom large, and must factor in to decisions about the future of the health care system. So while excellence must be maintained, excess should be removed."[19] Excess is, of course, in the eye of the beholder. What is "excess" to a bureaucrat is a life-saving procedure to a sick person.

The French insistence to stick with the fairness doctrine while not addressing the real cause of runaway costs – over-utilization from entitlement thinking – holds the danger of a costly slide into medical mediocrity. Hopeful-

18. Ibid., 4.
19. See note 1, 3.

ly, they will never again suffer a heat wave or other national disaster that will cost thousands of lives.

Nowhere, though, is the fairness doctrine more ingrained than in Germany, the grandparent of all socialist health care systems.

CHAPTER 19
SOLIDARITY IN THE
MOST MATURE SYSTEM:
GERMAN HEALTH CARE

Germany's 82 million citizens live in a country of 137,850 square miles, smaller than California. Germany spends $260 billion, 11.1 percent of its $2.36 trillion GDP on health care.

Germany offers a very mature government-controlled health care system and holds to idealistic standards. Germany, however, is beset by the same cost problems faced by every modern country.

Germany's GDP has slipped during the last few years, as has its total workforce, with unemployment stuck above 10 percent. (U.S. unemployment generally is in the 5 to 6 percent range.) One of Germany's chronic problems is the high cost of labor, and this is driven in part by its generous employee benefits programs, including health coverage.

Germany is the world's pioneer in socialist health care systems. The first formal state-imposed system began in 1883 when the government mandated health insurance coverage for certain employee classes. Employees and their employers funded the insurance. Thus began the Bismarck System of social security that eventually included coverage for disability, old age, unemployment, and long-term health care.

From its inception, several operating principles have defined the German system:

> 1) "...social solidarity,
> 2) insurance premiums for the sickness funds are a proportional payroll tax,
> 3) free choice of a physician as well as nearly full coverage for all services,
> 4) higher-income people may opt out of the system and buy private health insurance,
> 5) obligatory insurance for all employees with an income lower than a certain level,
> 6) definition of the benefit package in self-administration by a committee of sickness funds and health care providers..."[1]

The key to the German system is social solidarity, meaning socialism. Germans stubbornly cling to this principle, and it costs them dearly.

Those early mandatory health benefits programs required employees to pay two-thirds of the insurance cost, while employers paid the rest. The national government wrote the controlling laws, but left it to the German states to administer and regulate the insurance funds.

EVOLUTION OF GERMAN HEALTH CARE BENEFITS

Employers were required to pay 100 percent of the cost of accident funds (similar to America's workers compensation insurance) for their workers. This is one reason that

---

1. Prof. Dr. J.-Matthias Graf von der Schulenburg, "German Health Care System in Transition, The difficult way to balance Cost Containment and Solidarity," *European Journal of Health Economics*, 2005.

even today, the German health care system pays for care at a health spa, since employers believed that such a lavish benefit would help their employees to return to work much sooner.

Eventually, the government mandated health insurance for more worker categories. The system evolved from one where workers first paid their own bills and then submitted a reimbursement request, to a program where insurance companies directly paid for medical services, which removed the worker from any financial responsibility. The patient used services without knowing or caring about their cost.

Perhaps recognizing the limits of their socialist system to provide everyone with needed services, "Germany is the only [European] country, where high-income people, self-employed and civil servants may opt out of the compulsory social security scheme and join private health insurance."[2]

DOCTOR POWER AND GROWTH OF THE SYSTEM

By 1920, doctors' unions represented 75 percent of German doctors, and the government included them on their insurance regulatory panels. Doctors used work slowdowns and strikes when necessary to win concessions from insurance funds. Primary care doctors held iron-grip power over the system

During the extreme financial crisis of the Weimar Republic in the 1920s, revenue in the sickness funds shrank, but the consumption of health care increased. To control the cost of health care, the government began requiring workers to make co-payments.

---

2. See note 1, 2.

NAZI HEALTH CARE INCREASED SOCIALIZATION

During Hitler's rule, the Nazi government advanced socialized health care, extending sickness fund benefits to retired persons and hospital coverage to dependents. The Nazis, however, refused to provide insurance coverage for Jews and other oppressed minorities, though it required all laborers to help pay the bills. This is graphic evidence that a system run by a government always has the potential to discriminate, whether based on selected diseases it no longer wants to cover, or against political minorities or ethnic groups it dislikes.

After World War II, France, the United Kingdom, the United States, and Russia each tried to establish their own health care system preferences in the new Germany. The U.S. tried to institute market-based care, while the others tried various forms of socialized medicine.

The Russians imposed a communist health care system on East Germany. "However, due to under-financing, [by the late 1980s] personnel shortages and lack of access to modern equipment, the GDR [East German] health care system gradually began to fall behind the standards of western industrialized countries..."[3] Not until after the fall of the Berlin Wall did East Germany's health care system begin to catch up with the modern world.

GERMAN ECONOMY STRUGGLES FROM HIGH COSTS; STILL, SOCIALISM EXPANDS THE SYSTEM

By 1955 the pre-war health care system had been restored, with sickness funds and primary care funded by employers and employees. Employers alone funded injury

---

3. Reinhard Busse and Annette Riesberg, "Health Care Systems in Transition," World Health Organization, 2004, 22.

and disability insurance. These generous benefit costs, now locked in place, became a competitive burden for German industry, often making their products too expensive in foreign countries – today, they still struggle to be competitive in world markets.

During the late 1960s and into the 1970s, German health care authorities replaced religiously-based health care providers with secular operations. This meant increased costs for the publicly-financed system.

Technology, medical advances, and access to more care all put increasing upward pressure on spending. Germany could not isolate itself from pricing problems experienced in other modern nations.

Despite cost pressures, the government expanded mandatory coverage to farmers, disabled persons, and students. More patients were now consuming more medical care at a time when technology had begun to drive up spending. (During this time period, the U.S. Congress had created a similar dilemma through Medicare, Medicaid, and the new HMO programs that it had come to favor.)

In 1972, the German government shifted some structural health care costs away from funding by health insurance. It did this by requiring state governments to pay for investments in hospitals and clinics. Governments, then, bought and paid for medical facilities, transferring their funding away from insurance premiums and onto taxation.

Germany tried health care competition, but burdened it with so many requirements that it did nothing to hold down costs. "German sickness funds compete against each other. However, due to the identical definition of the benefit catalogue by the joint committee, this competition is limited, did not work well, and means primarily that members may switch from one fund to another every year for lower contribution rates."[4] Germans did what people everywhere always do, gravitating to where they could purchase the most insurance for the least cost.

THE FALL OF THE WALL

In 1990, after the fall of the Berlin Wall, and the beginning of reunification of East and West Germany, the country faced a health care challenge unlike all other nations. East Germany's communist health care system had to merge with Germany's government-controlled system. Where the communist system relied entirely on public ownership and funding, the socialist German system relied on a combination of government taxes and employer /employee paid private insurance.

Germans instituted mandatory long-term health insurance as a way to deal with their aging population. This created an additional tax and funding burden for their citizens. By 1996, German health care managers were forced to increase co-payments, but ration preventive and rehabilitative services. Cost realities forced them to drop some benefits, including the loss of paid dental care for children.

In 1997, the government passed the Health Insurance Cost-Containment Act, a law designed to force increased cost controls on providers and restrain the increases in insurance costs.[5] All future increases in the payment of benefits were to be tied to increases in Germans' income, hoping this would keep their economy competitive with those of other European nations. Productive economies, however, do not work in this manner. Imposing price and supply controls means nothing if there is an outbreak of disease or, on the other hand, a couple of very healthy

4. See note 1, 2.
5. See note 3, 24.

years. As all of us know too well, the human body ignores government planning (or even our planning), getting sick at the most inopportune times. This is one of the main reasons why centrally-planned health care systems always fail to meet their citizens' needs.

When a new government formed in 1998 made up of a coalition of the Social Democratic Party and the far-left Green Party, the health care system moved to expand coverage once again. (The German ruling coalition was popularly labeled the Reds and the Greens.) Some of the 1996 exclusions were reinstated. The new government placed stringent cost controls in place, forcing providers to abide by government pricing methods.

The Reds' and Greens' answer to the failures of their socialist system was to try to increase its socialist programs. Such a strategy proved politically popular for a short time, but both parties lost heavily during the 2005 elections.[6] Germany's politics had become somewhat more conservative.

CONTROL OF HEALTH CARE AND DELIVERY OF SERVICES

Germany's 16 states have very little say in health policy, other than regulating and planning local health care entities. This removes major health care decisions from each German citizen while placing overall responsibility in the national government. Citizens express their pleasure or ill will at election time, but ultimately will bear the cost of the system through taxes, co-payments, lower income, higher unemployment, and rationing, with very little recourse. It is hard to appeal to a national health care gov-

---

6. "September 18, 2005 Bundestag Election Final Results – Federal Republic of Germany Totals," Election Resources on the Internet: Elections to the German Bundestag - Results Lookup, http://electionresources.org/de/bundestag.php?election=2005

erning body, given its sheer size and political distance from individual patients.

During the 2005 campaign debate about German health care reform, the Reds and Greens offered the "People's Insurance Scheme." Their plan would have eliminated private insurance altogether.[7] Perhaps this contributed to their election losses.

The minority party had its own plan. It required a flat fee per person, except that poor people would be subsidized through general taxes. Government would pay the insurance costs of children. This system would result in massive cost shifting, transferring much of the costs to Germany's eldest citizens. "The elderly population would have to bear a greater share of health care costs and ... capital would be saved by the young age groups or by all members of the social and private health insurance funds."[8] This is the reverse of what has happened in America, where working people and taxpayers underwrite the costs of Medicare, and all taxpayers underwrite the cost of health care for the poor. In Germany, generational warfare has already broken out.

Is the End of Solidarity In Sight?

Both the majority and minority parties believed that the way to fund health care reform was to shift its entire cost to employees. By relieving the employers from paying these costs they hope that individuals will earn more, and German products will become more competitive in worldwide markets. Still, they admit that these schemes will not control spiralling health care costs.

We found that some German writers worry that recent

---

7. See note 1, 2.
8. Prof. Dr. Klaus-Dirk Henke, Prof. Robert F. Rich, Prof. Dr. Hilmar Stolte, M.D., "Lessons Learned From Other Health Care Systems," Technische Universitat Berlin, Nov. 2004, 14.

reforms might spell the end of the Bismarckian health insurance system. "It is most likely that competition among sickness funds will exist only on paper, and national health insurance will be the result,"[9] wrote Professor Dr. J. Matthias Graf von der Schulenburg as early as 1994.

In many ways, the Germans stand at the same crossroad as we do in the United States. Either the health care system will need to move toward more free market solutions, or to a total state takeover. Germany's dilemma is worse than ours, however, in that they have tried the state system for more than 120 years, and despite finding that it fails them, still stubbornly cling to the fairness principle – solidarity – that stifles market forces from correcting their financial ills. They see that everyone is in the same boat, and so, deserve equal access to affordable health care.[10] The world watches as their boat slowly sinks, stung by high costs, high utilization, and a declining German population.

Costs continue to be driven higher by an aging population, technology, and demand for more and higher quality care. Co-payments were increased again in January 2004 in another effort to hold down overall costs, causing the government to put caps on total payments, establishing global budgeting. Global budgeting, we have seen in other countries, inevitably results in long waiting lines and rationing.

HOSPITALS SEARCH FOR SOLVENCY AND SOLUTIONS

Hospitals find that they are better off if they specialize, but the government does not like this as it creates a form of social and financial discrimination. To counteract this trend

---

9. Prof. Dr. J. Matthias Graf von der Schulenburg, "The German Health Care System at the Crossroads," *Health Economics, Vol. 3,* 1994, 3.
10. "Terminating stagnation – redesigning the system," German Association of Research-Based Pharmaceutical Companies, 2005, http://www.vfa.de/en/articles/art_2002-02_001.html

(with some exceptions), after 2005, each hospital now has to show that they perform a minimum number of each kind of procedure. "For instance, if a hospital does not conduct more than a certain number of liver transplants per year it will not receive payments for knee operations."[11] Such a policy could create rather bizarre marketing programs as hospitals try to attract specific individuals with the maladies needed by the hospital to provide surgical balance.

Dr. Dirk-Henke, of the Technische Universität in Berlin, suggests, "...[I]t would certainly be advantageous if insurers had their own hospitals, primary care facilities and rehabilitation as well as all services needed for comprehensive coverage."[12] In the U.S., many state governments are seeking to split up these sorts of business relationships, having learned that when the payer and the provider are the same, the patient can come out a distant third.

The German system has tried to introduce managed care procedures since 1997, and even now implements evidence-based medicine standards, though it admits that the reforms have not worked very well.

Starting in 2005, specialists will be paid based on the cost of care for certain types of diseases, with the government instituting strict budget caps on each group and doctor. In this way, they will be encouraged to not practice too much medicine – rationing health care.

LESSON LEARNED: MIXED SYSTEMS DO NOT WORK SO WELL

When reforms forced doctors to assume control over the overall cost of drugs, "doctors responded by making

---

11. See note 1.
12. See note 8.

additional referrals to specialists and hospitals (who were not subjected to limits), which cost an estimated 1.4 billion DM [Deutsche Marks]."[13] This caused J. Matthias Graf von der Schulenburg, writing in the *European Journal of Health Economics*, to conclude that mixed systems don't work well: that is, when part is government controlled and part is market driven, then governments have to try to impose more regulations and controls on providers and patients. (It is hard to avoid the obvious; this is precisely what happened following the United States' introduction of Medicare, Medicaid, and the old forms of rigid, closed-ended staff HMOs.)

German health care leaders know that they must find a solution to hold down runaway spending. They turn to modest market-based solutions while refusing to address the real problem: "In Germany health care services are zero-priced, leading to excess demand," Dr. Felder wrote. "Co-payments represent the best remedy for this problem."[14] He adds, "[S]ociety pays a high price if it provides health care services for free."[15] Centralized, nationalized health care has left them hamstrung for real solutions.

The frustrations currently faced by Germans may be seen in this quote: "Higher out-of-pocket payments and rationing of services can lower utilization and cost but are seen in contradiction with the solidarity goal, sacrosanct in social policy in Germany. To combine competition and rationing with the solidarity principle is still an unsolved challenge for German's health politicians, as competition needs and leads to inequality, while solidarity calls for equal access to medical services for everyone."[16]

---

13. See note 9.
14. Prof. Dr. Stefan Felder, "Reform of Germany's Health Care Market," Institute of Social Medicine and Health Economics, University of Magdeburg, Germany, Maritim ProArte Hotel, Berlin, revised version July 4, 2002
15. Ibid.
16. See note 1, 10.

WILL IT ALL WORK?

The world's view of German health care quality has been slipping. "Quality improvement became a dominant political issue after the publication of international comparative studies showing the relatively low performance of the German health care system."[17]

Instead of being the envy of the world, the WHO said in 2000 that German health care had slipped to number 13. Sandwiched between France's number one rating and Germany's number 13, are such tiny countries as San Marino, Andorra, and Malta. The WHO's view of German health care is blurred by the country's reliance on private health insurance, and allowing some wealthier people to purchase private care, a bit too much of the free market for the World Health Organization.

So what is Germany's response to this criticism? "The reaction to this gap between performance and cost of medical care is massive governmental regulation and intervention to increase quality of care...,"[18] and this they attempted by creating yet another government agency charged with improving the system.

The European Union will most likely attempt to force other reforms onto the German system, and some of those reforms may be profound. These, too, will affect the United Kingdom, France, and other E.U. nations, perhaps reshaping their health care systems by further centralizing the determination of benefits and costs of health insurance.

---

17. Ibid., 8.
18. Ibid., 9.

CHAPTER 20
EUROPE'S FAIRNESS DOCTRINE CONFRONTED BY MARKET FORCES

Health care systems everywhere are reeling from the effects of rapidly increased spending. European (and Canadian) governments with their strict central government controls are not immune from this problem. They have tried to meet the challenge by rationing services, reducing the number of physicians, reducing access to technology, or as a sort of last resort, turning to some forms of free market devices. For instance, "Spain and Italy are in the process of decentralizing policy and finance to regions."[1] Decentralization means moving toward the break up of the federal government monopoly.

People everywhere want to live longer and healthier lives, and they want others to help pay their bills. Europe's problems are made worse because of their stubborn allegiance to the fairness doctrine. So they face "...the growing challenges of restraining costs, improving quality and assuring universal access [which] have put the health systems of Europe under severe pressure."[2]

---

1. Peter C. Smith, "Health care reforms in Europe and their implications for Japan," *The Japanese Journal of Social Security Policy: Vol. 3, No. 2*, Dec. 2004, 80.
2. Ibid.

Most nations are resorting to co-payments to slow down health care spending. They have come to understand that patients need to have at least some money at risk when they see a doctor. Sweden, a nation known for cradle-to-grave social services, now requires a co-payment. The Netherlands recently began moving in that direction, as did Italy. Yet, health care managers fret because "the impact of these co-payments is abated by a flourishing market in voluntary complementary health insurance," used by many citizens to pay these additional costs.[3] This shows that when they are given a choice to spend more of their own money, European citizens understand the value of voluntary health insurance.

Some of the countries with health plans that pay for prescription drugs have created a system of "reference pricing," in which they set reimbursement rates for families of drugs, and any costs above that must be paid by the patient. In so doing, they hope to encourage people to buy generic drugs, which are far less expensive than name brand drugs.

The European socialists systems have also begun to recognize that competition between hospitals, clinics, and doctors will help restrain costs while increasing quality. Unfortunately, the governments have left a heavy burden of regulation in place and therefore "have never been allowed to work in the way that a true market would function."[4]

In England and the Netherlands, the governments have granted operational freedom to some publicly-owned health facilities, and are "...encouraging market entry of for-profit providers, and...privatizing some providers."[5]

Other market reforms include allowing insured persons to buy insurance from the company of their choice, provid-

3. Ibid., 83.
4. Ibid., 85.
5. Ibid., 86.

ing increased information about doctors and hospitals, and imposing practice guidelines on doctors.

The European systems have struggled to provide consistent quality. "...[T]here is a growing awareness that there is a serious problem of major shortcomings in effectiveness, in the form of the quality of health care..."[6] In the past, quality issues "have been largely ignored."[7] To improve quality, the Europeans have turned to working with the providers to improve care, and attempting to give patients more choices, but this has created a new problem. Patient choice, the Europeans are learning, increases demand for more and better services, and that requires even more health care spending. Since so much of the cost of health care must be paid from taxes, and since their economies have been stagnant, or in decline, this has made it even more difficult to meet their citizens' health care demands.

To encourage choices, but hold down costs, the Europeans are toying with a unique idea to serve the needs of chronically ill patients. "...[O]nce a patient's needs have been assessed, the patient can be awarded a cash sum with which to purchase health care...This would effectively introduce a 'voucher' scheme for some aspects of chronic care."[8] Such a notion sounds like the kind of free market approach that the U.S. should consider.

Yet the greatest impediment to true cost containment while increasing quality is, that "...*voluntary health insurance run[s] the risk of compromising European principles of solidarity and fair access to health care.*"[9] [Emphasis added.] The idea that citizens should be free to decide whether to own health insurance, or to purchase the type of

6. Ibid., 88.
7. Ibid., 89.
8. Ibid., 90.
9. Ibid., 91.

insurance that best meets their need, violates the fairness doctrine, and the fairness doctrine is the foundation of all socialist systems.

In the United States, we tend to embrace the idea that everyone should be able to receive health care. We are, however, spared the economic damage done by socialist systems controlled by the fairness doctrine, recognizing that free-will, competition, and a culture of work will provide everyone with more and better health care. We have, at least until now, still held quite stubbornly to a free market doctrine.

WHAT CONCLUSIONS, THEN?

At the beginning of chapter 14 we asked, "Aren't there many health care systems in the world that are superior to ours? Shouldn't we be reforming our system to look like theirs?" The answer is no. Other health care systems are not superior; many are adopting market reforms.

Foreign health care systems that are controlled by government planners leave patients to needlessly suffer in long waiting lines. Health care is rationed by official government policy, putting politicians and bureaucrats in charge rather than citizens. The appearance that health care is free increases utilization and overall costs. These foreign economies do not generate the amount of wealth needed to be able to provide more health care services to their people. They spend 10 percent or less of their GDP on health care because it is all they can afford. We may complain about spending 15.3 percent of our GDP on health care, but we do it because we can, and the whole world benefits as a result.

What really sticks out when we do an honest appraisal

of other systems is that most of them have shown that a government-run system, without free market choices, does not meet their citizens' needs. Most countries have turned to a form of privately paid insurance, and in the case of Canada, send many of their sickest patients to America.

Every nation faces increased spending, all populations are aging, and wherever government controls the delivery of health care, the problems get more complicated and expensive. Whenever citizens are free to consume unlimited health care services paid for by others, use will go up, waste will increase, problems will compound, and prices will soar.

CHAPTER 21
THE HARD QUESTIONS THAT DEMAND ANSWERS AT THE FORK IN THE ROAD

"When you come to the fork in the road, take it."
Yogi Berra
Hall of Fame Professional Baseball Catcher and Manager

The United States' health care system stands at a fork in the road. Unlike Yogi's advice, however, we actually have to make a choice to go to the left, or the right.

For the past 40 years, Americans have come to believe that they are entitled to unlimited health care benefits paid for by others. As a result, the cost of health care continues to spiral higher. These accelerating costs can be used to frighten us in an effort to move us toward a government takeover of health care. We are told that the government can provide health care for less cost, yet still deliver higher quality services than the free market can.

Those who tell you to choose a government-run monopoly system have predicted "...collapse [of private health care] and for federal intervention to take place somewhere between 2008 and 2012."[1] So, which road do you think we should take?

CANNOT HAVE IT BOTH WAYS

The truth is that the U.S. health care system has already completed Phase I on the road toward becoming a socialized health care system. These are the signs:

> The costs of health care services are unknown to its users, so services are perceived to be free or almost free.
>
> People believe that health care is an inalienable right like life, liberty, and the pursuit of happiness.
>
> Since health care is a right, everyone is entitled to it.
>
> Everyone is entitled to have others help pay for their health care, even if they refuse to insure themselves.

Should we move toward Phase II of the socialization process, as those who favor a government-run system desire? In Phase II we tell the government to create a new system that they manage, because we cannot trust ourselves or private interests.

If we choose Phase II, we do it knowing that we are asking the government to make the hard decisions about who will get what care, and how much. It will mean turning our heads away so as not to see when "other people" are denied care; it must happen because the government will have to cut some services to hold down spending.

---

1. Richard L. Reece, M.D. *Voices of Health Reform, Options for Repackaging U.S.Health Care,* Practice Support Resources, Inc., 2005, 204.

266

Even as we look away, we will believe that our own needs will always be met. We will, however, be dead wrong. Eventually, we will all be one of the "other people."

So, as we stand at the fork in the road, this is the precise choice we are making: whether to move from Phase I to Phase II in the socialization process, or to release the power of the free market to cure health care.

Those who want us to choose a federal government takeover of health care have made many claims. It's time for us to ask them several hard questions. We believe they must answer these questions to convince us to choose Phase II.

The overarching question: Is it true that a socialized, government monopoly health care system will cost less, while delivering a greater abundance of higher quality services than the free market can?

THE NECESSARY QUESTIONS

Question: Why is the average annual cost of care for enrollees in government Medicaid programs so high, at $7,490[2] per person per year? Why is it even more than the cost for seniors on Medicare (at $7,061)?[3] Why is it nearly 250 percent greater than those with private health insurance (at $3,088)?[4]

We know that Medicaid pays for nursing home care for low-income seniors. Even accounting for the high cost of nursing home care, average spending for Medicaid patients

---

2. According to the Centers for Medicare and Medicaid Services (CMS), state and federal governments spent $267 billion for Medicaid services during 2003. Table HI-1, provided by CMS, states that 35.6 million people were served by Medicaid during 2003. $267 billion divided by 35.6 million is $7,490.
3. "Table 12: Per Enrollee, Expenditures and Growth in Medicare Spending and in Private Health Insurance Premiums, Calendar Years 1969-2003," indicates that private health insurance paid an average of $3,088 in claims during 2003.
4. Ibid., indicates that private health insurance paid an average of $3,088 in claims during 2003.

is $6,363,[5] or more than $25,000 for a family of four. Maybe this high cost is the result of caring for those with severe disabilities, but there surely are not 34 million of them.

Do people on Medicaid require more care, and if so, why? Are some taking advantage of the program by using more services than necessary, because they are "free"? Or, is the Medicaid system overrun by bureaucratic waste, program overlap, and inefficiencies?

GOVERNMENT ADMINISTRATIVE COST

Question: How much of the $766 billion in taxes we paid in 2003 to provide government health care services was spent on administrative expense?

The government tells us that its overall administrative costs were 4.8 percent compared to 9.9 percent for private insurance companies.[6] The authors believe that government administrative costs are really far greater than this. We discovered that a great deal of administrative cost is buried in other categories of state and federal budgets, though it is impossible for us to tally.

For instance, one spending item is titled, "Public Health Activities."[7] These include the costs of "...spending by governments to organize and deliver health services and to prevent or control health problems."[8] And, "State and local government public health activity expenditures are

---

5. According to the Abstract of the United States, Table 133, for the period ending 2000, there are 1.7 million Medicaid nursing home patients. Table 125 of the US Abstract states that $51 billion was spent to provide care for those 1.7 million people. Factoring out these numbers and costs means that Medicaid health care for 33.9 million people cost state and federal governments $216 billion, or $6,363 each.
6. "Table 3: National Health Expenditures, by Source of Funds and Type of Expenditure: Selected Calendar Years 1998-2003," Centers for Medicare and Medicaid.
7. Ibid. It is a line item near the bottom of the table, and is listed as an expense for each year reported.
8. "National Health Expenditures Accounts: Definitions, Sources, and Methods Used in the NHEA 2004," Centers for Medicare and Medicaid, 4.

primarily for the operation of State and local health departments."[9] This certainly sounds like administrative cost, but the government counts it as a different kind of expense. We think an honest comparison requires defining a good part of these expenses as administrative cost, since they represent nearly 21 percent – $46.3 billion – of state and local health care spending.[10] What we know for sure is that this money does not get to doctors and hospitals to provide health services to patients.

We know that private insurance companies must pay the expenses of owning and operating office buildings and supporting staff work. These are administrative costs. Do state and federal governments include these costs as administrative expense? Or are these costs paid under some other expense category unrelated to health care?

Private insurance companies pay for the marketing and selling of their products and services to clients. Governments use caseworkers to manage their health care programs, to identify, explain and deliver services. Does the government count the cost of employing these people as administrative expense?

Insurance companies are forced by law to pay premium, Medicaid and HMO taxes, and other assessments. They report these as administrative cost and run more than five percent.[11] Governments have no such expenses, making it appear that they can do more work for less cost.

Federal and state government budgets are massive. We contend that no one, in or out of government, can provide an honest, accurate accounting of the true administrative costs of government-run health care. So we ask those who favor a national health care system to prove any savings in

---

9. Ibid., 15.
10. See note 6.
11. Actual quote prepared for a client, provided by Health Partners to Dattilo Cons., Inc., disclosing the various costs involved in calculating group insurance rates, Feb. 17, 2006.

administrative cost, and to assure us that those costs will not just be shifted to other government budget line items.

HERE'S A WAY TO PROVE YOU ARE RIGHT

Question: Why not combine Medicaid and all the other special health care programs into one big national government system, and let Washington, D.C. show us what it can do? Since 77 million people already receive their health care through these programs, combining them all into one single-payer system would be a good test of whether the government really can deliver better health care more efficiently.

Combine Medicare, Medicaid, Community Health Centers, state-based insurance programs and all the rest into one, cost-effective package. This would demonstrate whether a national health care system would save tens of billions of dollars in administrative expenses.

BUT YOU MIGHT FIRST HAVE
TO TRIM GOVERNMENT BENEFITS

Question: Why does group health insurance for government employees cost so much more than private, non-government employees? We learned, "...in September 2004, the average cost per public-sector employee per hour worked was $3.49 for health insurance, compared to $1.56 per hour worked for private-sector workers."[12]

Why does it cost the government 224 percent more than private free market employers to provide health benefits to their employees? Government employees are a cross-section of Americans, and would have the same health profile as the rest of us. So why does it cost so much

---

12. "State/Local Government Pay & Benefits Much Higher Than in Private Sector, But Jobs, Skills Differ," Employee Benefit Research Institute, April 6, 2005.

more to insure them compared to private, non-government employees?

Today, private employers insure 2.25 employees for the same cost as one government employee. Wouldn't it make sense for governments to adopt private employers' health insurance programs, and save tens of billions of tax dollars? Why would we want to go the other way, and increase private employers' cost by 225 percent?

WHICH FOREIGN SYSTEM WOULD YOU CHOOSE AS A MODEL?

Question: Can anyone name a modern foreign government monopoly health care system that has controlled spending without rationing, or without turning to some form of private insurance? Can anyone show such a system that has solved the problem of escalating health care costs without cutting services to citizens?

ADDRESSING FAIRNESS

Question: In a U.S. national health care system, how much emphasis will be placed on the fairness doctrine? Would we still be free to spend our own money, as much as we want and where we want, to purchase health care services to save our child's or spouse's life?

If the answer is "yes," then the first rule of the fairness doctrine has been violated. It would mean that some people could get more than other people, and that would be unfair. If the answer is "no," it suggests that a legal prohibition must be placed on private health care expenditures. Who would enforce that limit, and how?

Those who favor a federal takeover of health care are committed to the fairness doctrine. They call it equal access to affordable health care. The fairness doctrine prohibits the use of discretionary income to purchase more or better health care services by any individual. Yet, people faced with the death of a child or spouse will always want to spend their own money if it will help. Someone will have to say "no" to them. In a national health care system, would that be a federal bureaucrat?

ACCEPTABLE LEVEL OF CARE

Question: Reducing the cost of services and cutting overall spending on health care would be the most compelling reasons to give control to the government. So we want to know, what quality and quantity of care could we expect from a government-run system?

The European solidarity principle has resulted in waiting lines, technology and physician shortages, unnecessary death, and the inability to respond quickly to public health problems. How will the U.S. government resolve the common problem that these other countries face as they discriminate against sick people, as they deny care to the sickest and most vulnerable of their population. Is that what the U.S. would do?

We learned that determining "the appropriateness of medical care"[13] is one of the most important functions of a national health care system. Would a U.S. national system use this same logic? We wonder about this because H.R. 3600, the 1994 health care bill, specified it.

If a national council decides that some type of health care treatment is inappropriate, would that treatment be abandoned, even if it was saving a life, or reducing chronic suffering?

It is illegal in some foreign countries to purchase health

---

13. H.R. 3600, 103rd Congress, line 10, 848.

care services outside of the national system. This leaves the options of preparing for death, or dealing with a life of pain and suffering. As the British say, "We shall never have all we need...Expectations will always exceed capacity."[14]

If you say, "Oh, that will never happen in the United States," then how else will the government managers cut cost and spending?

CUTTING DOCS TO CUT COST?

Questions: Will the number of available doctors be reduced to control health care spending? How can the government make sure that there will be enough critical care specialists at the time and place they are needed most?

The 1994 proposed health care law declared that the number of doctors "shall be reduced..."[15] Those who wrote that language believed it had to be done to reduce health care spending. The bill even specified that it would pay medical schools more than $23 billion not to train doctors.[16] Is that how a new U.S. government-run health care system will work?

WHO GUIDES THE DOCS?

In a new, government-run health care system, who will create and enforce practice guidelines on doctors? Practice guidelines, we are told, are designed to help doctors choose the best and most efficient (least expensive) strategy to treat medical problems.

A lot has been said about physician groups creating their own practice guidelines. This is often called evidence-

---

14. "About the NHS, Balancing Demands," http://www.nhs.uk/england/abouthenhs/history/1948to1957.cmsx.
15. See note 13, lines 9-11, 513.
16. See note 13, lines 8-15, 519.

based, science-based medicine, or health outcomes. Doctors know much more about doctoring than do bureaucrats and lawyers. If doctors and medical scientists develop practice guidelines, we might have a greater level of comfort than if government bureaucrats design them.

What makes us nervous is that the 1994 proposed law said, "The National Quality Management Council *shall direct the Administrator for Health Care Policy and Research to periodically review and update clinically relevant guidelines...*"[17] [Emphasis added.] That surely made us think that federal medical bureaucrats would be in charge. Are we right?

WHO WILL BE IN CHARGE?

Question: In a government-run system, who would have the ultimate control over our personal health care decisions? Would it be a national health care board, like in the 1994 health care bill? That law gave final power for health insurance rates, operating budgets, reimbursements, and a set of essential benefits to a national health board.[18] The president would appoint its 15 members, and none of them were to be common health care consumers. Is that what we should do in the United States?

The national health board, had this law passed, would have been so powerful that any variations from its policies required an act of Congress.

The national health board would have had the power to impose penalties of $10,000, $50,000, even $100,000 on those who violated its rules.[19] We would surely want to know, before letting the federal government take over

---

17. See note 13, lines 10-18, 847.
18. See note 13, 996-1018.
19. See note 13, 153, 712, 930.

health care, if this is the kind of control we would be giving to them, and whom they could punish.

MY PERSONAL HEALTH CARE

Question: If U.S. voters choose a government-run system, how much would the government need to know about the health issues of individual citizens? How would the government managers know the appropriate amount of money to spend on certain health conditions without obtaining volumes of private patient information?

H.R. 3600 gave the national health secretary the right to access all provider information in any form or manner the secretary deemed necessary.[20] In fact, the only way that the national secretary could make wise decisions would be to access and collect private health care data. How do we know that government planners wouldn't use this data to decide against treating certain kinds of diseases, like HIV/AIDS or those that attack specific ethnic groups, or decide against providing life support for premature babies, or seniors with Alzheimer's disease?

PAYING FOR HEALTH CARE
IN THE GOVERNMENT-RUN SYSTEM

Question: Who is going to pay the premiums and taxes needed to fund a government-run system? Will employers be forced to pay, no matter their company size or ability to do so? Will individuals be forced to pay, in the same manner as, say, the income tax is paid? Will we pay for all of our health care through taxes? Or will we pay taxes and be forced to pay for health insurance, too?

In Germany, employer-paid mandatory health insur-

---

20. See note 13, 1025-1026.

ance has been the law since 1883. Today, however, Germans debate about the wisdom of requiring individuals to pay their own premium, freeing up employers from that burden. How would you make this work when Germany, the grandfather of socialized health care, struggles with it?

The 1994 health care bill would have forced all employers – large, small, self-employed – to purchase health insurance for employees and their dependents. It required that companies would pay 80 percent of the premium cost.[21]

Even with all of its mandates, the writers of the 1994 law knew that a good number of people would remain uninsured.[22] Is it true that those who demand mandatory health insurance for everyone, already know that there will still be a great number of uninsured people?

WHO MAKES THE ULTIMATE DECISIONS?

Question: Who is going to decide which services to cover and which to refuse? How will you insulate health care decisions from political interests?

In the socialist, single-payer system, the ultimate decision about which services to offer is made by a committee. The committee may be politicians, elected and appointed, or it may be broader: a group of consumer advocates, providers, payers, and politicians. No matter how the committee is structured, it is subject to politics, because ultimately, its members are appointed by politicians.

How will you protect the general population from politically privileged people jumping to the front of the health care waiting line? How will you ensure that political

---

21. See note 13, 20, 1064.
22. See note 13, lines 11-13, 844.

friends won't get favors unavailable to common citizens? That would not be fair.

PROGRESS AND ADVANCEMENT OF MEDICAL CARE SERVICES

Question: Will you be able to ensure that medical research and technology breakthroughs will continue? Will the government take over all medical research?

The socialist, single-payer health care system operates under a global budget. This reduces the incentive for private individuals to risk money by investing in medical research.

If investors do decide to risk their own money, they will want assurances from national health care leaders that their new product or service will become a covered benefit in the government health care system. Does that mean they will have to buy political favor from politicians?

HOW MUCH TO CUT AND HOW MANY JOBS WILL BE LOST?

Question: How much should health care spending be cut? As a percentage of GDP, what spending level would be acceptable? Will it be the 7.7 percent of the UK, or the 11.1 percent of Germany? And how many jobs must be eliminated as a result of spending cuts? What kinds of jobs will be eliminated? Where? Which government board will determine whose job will be terminated?

When a global budget controls how much is available to be spent on health care, it places a limit on the number of health care related jobs it will support. It also limits spin-off jobs in the health care tapestry. To reduce costs, the socialized health care system has no choice but to reduce or limit the number of jobs.

Job creation is a direct result of how different people look at things. The socialist looks at a full glass and believes that it will overflow, so he shuts off the flow of water, and begins to siphon some of the water out – jobs are lost. The free market entrepreneur looks at a full glass and sees an opportunity to find a larger glass that only he can fill, creating more jobs.

The socialist rations services; the entrepreneur creates new services.

SO WHICH ROAD TO TAKE

The most extreme political liberals promote a centralized, single-payer health care system under total control of the government. More clearly, they support a socialist, government-run monopoly health care system.

They prefer a Canadian or European form of single-payer system, supported by taxes and mandatory health insurance. They have come to believe that only the government can effectively manage the massive and critical health care delivery system.

Most Americans believe that U.S. health care must be reformed. They, however, look to the free market to maximize personal choice, competition, and investment in new technology. They believe that individuals are capable of making their own choices. They want to limit the government's role, and protect the people against monopoly control, whether public or private.

Most Americans believe that the best health care is that which is managed, delivered, and paid for by those closest to the individual, not by a distant bureaucrat.

YOU SEE, IT REALLY IS YOUR CHOICE

Ultimately, whether the U.S. takes the left or right road depends on your choice. You will choose by how you purchase health care, and by whom you elect. You need to choose wisely, because your health matters!

So which road should we take? Should we enter Phase II and embrace a socialized health care system? Or, what might happen if we release the free market to meet our health care needs?

CHAPTER 22
CAN THE FREE MARKET CURE US?

Questions: What is the free market? How does it relate to health care? Can the free market eliminate waste, increase quality, and reduce health care costs? Can it solve the problems created by Phase I in the socialization process?

Defining a free market is to describe how it works. It is an "... economy based on supply and demand with little or no government control...where buyers and sellers are allowed to transact freely...based on a mutual agreement on price without state intervention in the form of taxes, subsidies or regulation."[1]

You are a shopper, and that makes you a key part of the free market. You clip coupons, watch advertisements, and head out to shop for the best value for your hard-earned dollar. You consider brands, sizes, quantities, quality and price. Then you make a purchase. That is the free market in action. Your spending choices are restrained by the limits

---

1. *The Free Dictionary*, by Farlex,
http://financialdictionary.thefreedictionary.com/Free+Market

of your income and assets, or your credit rating.

The free market works best when there are multiple choices of the same or similar products. These products compete with each other for your dollar. To be a successful shopper, you need ample, good information to know the price, quality, and whether the purchase will meet your needs and fit your budget.

FREE MARKETS MEAN CHOICES

Consider how you shop for a car. You have many choices. You can buy a compact, intermediate, or full size. It might be red, green, blue, or almost any color. There are scores of options from which to choose – DVDs, heated seats, power windows, and more. There are dozens of brand names, and each offer several models – sedans, convertibles, two-doors, four-doors, SUVs, pick-ups, minivans. The free market gives you many choices so you can buy exactly what you want.

If the government controlled the automobile industry as some think it should control health care, you would have one choice of a car and it would be a model designed to fit everyone. Although you would not pay for it out of your pocket (instead, by taxes), and you would not know its cost, you would be forced to own the car the government chose for you. The government model would be the one that politicians thought to be the most cost-effective, to try to hold taxes down. It would get you to where the government felt you ought to go, but if you are not happy with it, you would have no other choice but to complain to your elected representative.

FREE MARKETS VS. MONOPOLIES

The purpose of Monopoly, the board game, is for one

person to eliminate competition and control all the real estate, transportation and utilities. Then that person can take everyone else's money and win the game. In winning the game, however, everyone loses, even the person holding all the money, because there is no one left with whom to trade; the game is over.

Free markets and monopolies are like oil and water. They are not compatible, because competition is a key to the free market's success. When one business has a monopoly on a service or product, competition is stifled, individual choice is limited, cost goes up, and quality falls.

Again, let's consider cars. The old Soviet Union ran all industries as government monopolies. Competition was not allowed. They produced a car called the Yugo. Yugos survived in Russia, because there was no competition. Then importers brought the Yugo to the United States, where Americans had dozens of choices. It took but a short time for the Yugo to fail in the U.S. It could not compete in the free market. Why? Though they were inexpensive, they were also unreliable, and they lacked the options we wanted and for which we were willing to pay. We refused to buy them. Competition destroyed the Yugo.

Since our founding as a nation, U.S. citizens have told the government that we will not allow monopolies to function. Unfortunately, the government does not see itself as a monopoly, though it has total control of several critical aspects of life.

If the national government controlled U.S. health care, it would be a monopoly. It is a monopoly that should be strongly resisted, for all the same reasons that the government broke up the monopolies held by Standard Oil, AT&T, and Microsoft.

Monopolies of any kind destroy competition. Competition is essential to produce more and better options at a lower price than any monopoly system, whether it is public or private.

BREAKING UP MONOPOLIES

The federal government protects competition and encourages the free market by breaking up corporate monopolies. The AT&T breakup clearly demonstrates this principle.

Before 1974, consumers, in effect, had one choice for phone service: American Telephone & Telegraph (AT&T), through one of its wholly owned subsidiaries. There were also hundreds of small, independent local phone companies in operation, but AT&T was the Big Gorilla that dominated the business.

In those days, if you wanted telephone service, you did whatever AT&T demanded and paid whatever they asked (or what the government regulators allowed them to charge). You had one phone line. The phone company owned the telephones, so you paid a monthly rental charge for your rotary-dial phone; you could have any color you wanted as long as it was black. Many people had a party line, forced to share phone time with a neighbor. There were no added features, but you could call directory assistance as often as you liked at no extra charge. If you could afford a little more and wanted an extension, you could rent a second phone at additional cost.

When you made a long distance call, you had one choice: AT&T. Long distance rates often hit $2.00 a minute ($7.90 a minute in 2005 dollars).[2] You made long distance calls only for special purposes or emergencies, and kept the calls short.

---

2. Calculated using the United States Census Bureau "Inflation Calculator," at http://data.bls.gov/cgi-bin/cpicalc.pl

In 1974, the United States Justice Department filed suit to break up AT&T's monopoly. After the breakup, competition exploded.

Many companies entered the telephone business. Some of them already were large, successful corporations in related businesses, but a far greater number were tiny start-up companies whose future fortunes created wealth and jobs for millions of Americans. Competition – the drive to be the first, the most affordable, or the most unique – drove these new companies. The new services and products created by competition, however, went far beyond telephones. Communications technology also exploded.

As a result of competition, today's phone companies offer numerous features – call waiting, call forwarding, voice mail, caller ID, faxes, and more – at low cost, and you can choose from among dozens of phone styles and colors, even black. The internet and cell phones have become common, and this, too, is a result of telecommunications competition.

Without competition, the AT&T monopoly had no need to improve quality or create new products and services.

Nowhere are the benefits of competition more dramatic than with long distance rates. Long distance service today can be purchased at rates as low as three cents a minute. Some long distance providers charge a flat monthly fee for unlimited long distance calling. Many cell phone users pay nothing extra for long distance calls.

Everyone has benefited from the breakup of the AT&T monopoly and from the competition that followed. Today, nearly every American owns multiple telephones, and many have more than one phone number. Phone ownership cuts across all income levels; even low-income, poverty-level Americans have telephones. This is a result of free market competition replacing a government-regulated and protected monopoly.

WHAT DOES AT&T HAVE TO DO WITH HEALTH CARE?

You might argue that the health care system has little to do with telephone service, that they react differently to free market forces. We disagree.

What happened to long distance rates is similar to what happened to Claritin, the allergy medicine mentioned in chapter 10. Claritin's price had been protected by a temporary, legal monopoly through patent protection. At that time, it sold for about $900 a year. Insurance companies and government drug plans paid for the majority of Claritin prescriptions, shielding consumers from its true cost.

When the Federal Drug Administration approved Claritin as safe enough to be sold over-the-counter without a doctor's prescription, insurance no longer paid for it. Consumers had been used to paying a co-pay of $10 a month, and Claritin knew they had to drop the price to meet consumer expectations. They dropped the price to about $25 a month, from around $75 a month. The price of Claritin had dropped by more than 66 percent due to consumer pressure, not government price-setting. This shows how consumers acting together are far better at negotiating prices than the government or other third-party payers.

The free market, however, had not yet finished dealing with the price of Claritin. Once Claritin's patent protection had expired, competitors stepped in to offer alternatives. Eventually, Loradatine, a generic version of Claritin, became available over-the-counter at $14 a year, or less than $1.20 a month. The price of Claritin, thanks to the free market, had dropped more than 98 percent.

Low long distance rates and the price of Loradatine are

reflections of what the free market can do with products and services that consumers demand. And, they demonstrate the proper role of government, to break up destructive monopolies, and to provide patent protection for a limited amount of time.

HOW THE FREE MARKET REDUCES HEALTH CARE COST

You might wonder if the free market can actually deliver high quality health care at a reduced cost. Lasik surgery helps us see a clear picture of how this happens. Lasik surgery has helped tens of thousands of people throw away their glasses and see better than they have since childhood.

"In 1991 the first LASIK procedure was performed in the U.S."[3] Those earlier Lasik surgeries were offered by a handful of clinics and often cost as much as $10,000 per eye. As it became popular and was heavily promoted, more doctors offered the procedure, medical equipment prices fell, and the price of Lasik surgery dropped dramatically.

Today, "LasikPlus reported its average price per procedure in the fourth quarter of 2004 as $1,351" an eye.[4] Some Lasik providers advertise prices less than $600 or even $300 an eye.

This pricing process is totally consumer driven, because the patient pays 100 percent of the costs out of his or her own pocket. Lasik surgeons have had to set their prices at a level that their patients are willing to pay. This has reduced the cost of Lasik surgery so that it is accessible to almost everyone. It is a prime example of how the free market reacts to uninsured health services.

---

3. "History of Lasik Surgery," Philip Colenda, MD, PC, FAAO, http://www.westchestervision.com/historyoflasik.html.
4. Liz Segre, "Cost of Lasik and other corrective eye surgery," http://www.allaboutvision.com/visionsurgery/cost.htm

Another benefit that results from individuals paying the cost of Lasik is that it forces doctors to be efficient. They must make sure that they reduce waste so that their price can remain competitive and affordable.

The Lasik industry further adapted to the free market in much the same way as home builders, auto dealers, and major appliance stores have done. "In addition to competitive pricing, we have unequaled promotional financing options – extensive, flexible, convenient, and most with a $0 down payment," LasikPlus advertises.[5] If the patient cannot pay for the entire procedure before surgery, the Lasik provider arranges financing that provides affordable payments spread over a period of time.

SCANNING LOWER PRICES

Here is another example of how the free market lowers the cost of health care.

Medical inventors created numerous types of scanners that send sound or electronic impulses into and through a human body, so that a doctor can spot internal problems. Previously, a patient had to undergo dangerous and expensive exploratory surgery to receive the same results.

Free market competition took technology to the next level. In the last decade or so, heart scan clinics have offered a non-invasive procedure that allows doctors to see inside the human heart. The knowledge gained from the heart scan allows patients and doctors to design an exercise and medical plan to reduce the risk of a life-threatening condition. These procedures have always been affordably priced, and are generally not covered by insurance. In fact, because most individuals pay for their own heart scans, the

---

5. "At LasikPlus Vision Centers, All We Do is Perform Laser Vision Correction."
http://www.lasikplus.com/

price has dropped from $400 in 2000, to as little as $275 today, a reduction in price of more than 30 percent in five years.[6]

The government and health insurers pay for most other imaging scans, like MRIs and CAT scans. Their costs are far higher than the heart scan. An echogram, for instance, could cost $1,700 or more today.[7] If patients paid for their echograms directly, the cost would drop, as it has with heart scans and Lasik surgery.

People choosing to spend their own money on Lasik surgery or a heart scan control the price and availability of the procedure. As long as they do, the cost will tend to go down; that is the key to controlling health care spending.

There is, of course, a meeting place between paying all your own health care costs, and having someone else pay them for you. It is called catastrophic health insurance. Our parents and grandparents owned it, prior to Medicare.

Combined with what we now know after 40 years experience with the entitlement mentality, a new form of catastrophic insurance has the potential to solve the dual problems of paying for necessary health care, and restraining health care costs. Health care professionals and reformers call it "consumer-driven health care." It is the direction in which we ought to go to continue to receive the world's best health care at more affordable prices.

If we choose consumer-driven health care, the next chapter demonstrates what we can expect in the future, a future that is closer than you might think.

---

6. Via telephone call placed to Heartscan Minnesota, Jan. 26, 2006.
7. Prices based on estimate provided by the Heart Institute of the Cascades, for 2005, via email to the author on 11/21/05 and will vary depending on location, exact procedure and other factors.

Chapter 23
Tomorrow's Doctor Appointment

Tomorrow's health care system when compared to today, will be more exciting, more beneficial, save more lives, reduce more suffering, and give you more for your health care dollar – if you make the right choice.

By your vote, your personal choices, and your pocketbook, if you tell politicians, insurance companies, HMOs, and medical providers that you want a true free market, consumer-driven approach to health care, your doctor's appointment in the near future will go like this:

Recently you have noticed advertising for the Richman Clinic. You had also received their mailings, and saw their brochure in a rack at your primary care doctor's office.

You saw that the Richman Clinic was one of those new patient-centered clinics you had seen on TV news. That meant they used electronic medical records, they include you in making treatment decisions, you can know their charges in advance, and more. Their website gave you all their basic information and linked you to dozens of local health care choices. Your primary care doctor highly recommended Dr. Richman, too. And so, you decided to make an appointment.

"Hello. May I help you?" the smiling receptionist asks as you walk into the office.

"Yes, I have an appointment with Dr. Richman," you answer. "I made the appointment on your website last Monday."

"Yes, I see your name here."

"I saw on doctors.com that Dr. Richman's patients rate him highly. And it looks like he has experience with my condition," you explain.

"He's one of the best."

"I also noticed that your clinic's fees are affordable," you say, thinking about the fee information on the website.

"May I have your health care card, please?" the receptionist asks.

You hand her a plastic debit card with a magnetic strip on it, and she swipes it just as would a sales clerk. That card allows Dr. Richman's office to access your entire health record through an online connection. You enter your password on a keypad. As she swipes your card, it creates an electronic medical record on a portable notebook computer, opens a claim with your insurance company, and allows the receptionist to verify your current information.

You heard that Dr. Richman's fees were reduced during the last six months because new technology has made the clinic office system more efficient. Besides, there is a similar clinic just six blocks away, and you noticed that their fees were the same as the Richman Clinic's. It reminded you of how gas stations often sit across the street from each other, and their prices are almost always the same, or one is a few pennies lower.

One of the efficiencies that most pleases Dr. Richman and you is that he can see your entire medical history. That means he will not send you off to be prodded, scanned, and stuck needlessly for diagnostic tests you had recently. That, too, saves money. He also appreciates that by using your debit card, the clinic fee will be paid immediately after your office visit. That, too, has allowed him to charge lower fees.

Soon a nurse leads you to the exam room. She takes your temperature and blood pressure, and enters the information on the electronic notepad, then leaves the room. A few minutes later, a Physician's Assistant (PA) enters; she is a key member of the team of professionals who will deal with your needs.

"I see here that you had both lab tests done before you came today," the PA says, reading from your electronic record.

"Yes, when I got the email right after I made my appointment, it said to go to the lab on 10th Street and get these tests done. So I went last Thursday," you say, proud that you followed through on this.

"Thank you for doing that. It helps us all," she says, noticing that your electronic record indicates that your personal patient rating is very high. You are one of those cooperative patients that doctors love to see.

The PA conducts a preliminary examination and enters her findings on the electronic notepad. "Dr. Richman will be with you in a minute," she says, and then leaves the room.

While you wait, you look around the room. Its pastel walls and bright white tiled floor give it a feeling of life. You especially like the fact that it is spotlessly clean. A high window allows sunlight to flood the room. Even the magazines are this month's issues, and you choose one to page through while waiting. Everything about this room says, "You are welcome here. You are our valued patient."

Soon after, Dr. Richman enters the exam room. He reviews your health history, the preliminary exam, and lab test results. "Well, let me ask you a few questions," he begins.

He records your answers on the electronic notepad. When he is finished, he hits an enter key and within moments, a series of medical options appear on his screen. He prints out a copy for you so that you can look at them together. These options provide him with science-based guidelines to treat your condition. "These guidelines are developed by medical doctors in my specialty," he explains. "They have been tested and shown to produce the most successful outcomes for your condition."

"Sounds like a cake mix or something," you say, unsure that a computer program knows best how to solve your problem.

"Well put," Dr. Richman answers, chuckling softly. "They really are based on best science, but the good news is that, if I need to, I can deviate from them, if it's in your best interest. In the end, it's still my call. Well, actually, our call, because you're going to help me make that decision."

"Good, let's keep going," you say.

"Okay, here is what we're looking at," Dr. Richman begins, as he works through the information on your print-out with you. "Do you understand?" he asks at each step.

"Well, that makes it much clearer," you answer, looking at the notes you wrote on the printout. You are glad that the doctor doesn't have to rush out of the room.

"You can find more information about this here," Dr. Richman says, pointing at several website addresses printed on the bottom of the page. "You can also call this phone number and ask for CD number 2475, if you'd rather listen to the information. We even have a computer workstation just off the lobby, if you want to use our internet service. All this will help you further understand your situation. Okay?"

"Sounds good," you answer.

"Now let's choose the best option." Dr. Richman points at three drawings that appear on your printout. "If you choose surgery, it will go like this," he says, using the drawings to describe the procedure. He explains the surgical risks and the rewards.

"You may have read about Dr. Cutter who opened the new surgical center on Cedar Street," the doctor says.

"Yes, I remember a TV story about her," you answer. "She's kind of a high-tech surgeon."

"That's the one," Dr. Richman says. "If you choose surgery, you might want to consider her. She's worked with a national medical device company to develop new equipment that allows her to do a far less invasive procedure. It costs a little more, but you can go home the next day."

"I'd like that," you answer. "Just how much does the surgery cost?"

"The cost of this surgery will vary from about $9,000 to $12,000 for the hospital, plus the surgeon's fees," Dr. Richman explains. "So it depends on whom you choose, and of course, assuming there are no complications. Dr. Cutter's fees are higher than other surgeons, but the hospitalization costs are less."

"These are the three hospitals that do this kind of surgery, and here is Dr. Cutter's clinic," he says, pointing to the next page, right after the drawings, where there is a list of four medical providers. You notice the ratings for each provider printed in blue, right next to their listing.

"Thank you," you answer. You scratch your head and frown, saying "It is expensive. Will my insurance cover all the cost?"

"It looks like it," Dr. Richman answers after looking at the electronic notepad, "but make sure you check with your insurance company. I see that you have a $2,000 deductible policy."

"Okay," you say, knowing that you have saved more than that in your health savings account (HSA). Because your $2,000 deductible policy saved you thousands of dollars in premium during the last few years, you could afford to set aside money in your HSA. Though you had hoped to be able to keep some of that for retirement, you are glad it is there to offset the deductible.

"What are the other options?" you ask next.

"Many people get good results by following a drug regimen and doing a series of exercises," Dr. Richman says. Then he nods toward the computer screen, and together you view a short video that shows someone doing the exercises. They look like something you can do.

"And there's a need for weight loss: about 20 pounds," the doctor adds.

"Yes, I know," you sigh. "How much do the drugs cost?"

"There are about seven different drugs available. I would suggest this one, Xodium, for $92 a month," Dr. Richman says as he points to the printout, "or the generic version. It sells for about $30 at most drugstores. It's your choice. You will still have to pay those costs yourself until you use up your deductible, and you will have to stay on the drugs for at least six months before we will know if they're doing the job. You still might have to have the surgery after that."

"I see," you say. You are trying to picture yourself going through surgery and the thought makes you wince. "Well, I would prefer not having surgery unless it's really necessary. I'd rather try the drugs."

"That sounds like a good decision," Dr. Richman says, "but what about the exercises? If you don't do them, I think you'll have to have the surgery eventually."

"I understand," you say, rubbing your belly. "Well, I really don't want surgery, so I guess I'll have to exercise a bit, won't I?"

"Good," Dr. Richman says, "and that would save you more than a $1,000 on your deductible." He knows that if you are fully engaged in and committed to a health care regimen, you have a great chance of success.

Your session with Dr. Richman ends after 15 minutes. He leaves and a nurse comes in to finish entering the results of your visit into the electronic notepad. She also types in the prescription Dr. Richman wrote. "Do you still want this prescription to go to Neighborhood Drugs?" she asks. "That's what you had in your medical records."

"Yes, please."

"Oh, here's some good news. We have a 20 percent discount coupon for Neighborhood Drugs. I can attach that to the prescription." The nurse emails the prescription and the coupon to the drug store, and within minutes, the pharmacist has it filled, even before you have left the doctor's office.

The nurse shows you everything she has entered into the notepad. She also shows you the fee for your office visit that day.

"Is there anyone else who you would like us to send this information to," the nurse asks, "like a friend or family member?"

"Oh yes, please send it to my daughter. Here's her email address," you answer.

After you have read the information and verified the different services and prices that you just received, you sign the electronic notepad where it says, "I acknowledge that I received the above referenced medical services on this date, and authorize the payment of any and all claims for these services." When you press the enter key, the bank that handles your HSA immediately transfers funds to the Richman Clinic. An email is sent to your home summarizing your visit, to your primary care doctor, and to your daughter, as you requested.

"Now anytime you want to go over this, you can go to your health records at this internet address," the nurse says, pointing at your printout. "And remember that you can research all this other information about your condition at these other sites," she adds.

Before leaving, the nurse schedules a follow-up appointment for you with Dr. Richman. She also schedules a second appointment to be completed by telephone, so she can make sure that you have no further questions. "And I will ask you how your exercise program is going," she warns. "You should go to your medical record on the website each day as you exercise, and check off each exercise to keep track of how you are doing."

When you leave a few minutes later, you feel good about the time spent with the medical team at Richman Clinic. You now have a protocol to follow that you helped to choose, and you feel the costs are fair – you are getting your money's worth. You are glad that your insurance policy will cover future needs, and that today's bill has already been paid out of your HSA. You don't have to worry about losing your home, investments, or savings – your catastrophic health insurance makes them secure.

As you walk to your car, you think back to just a few years earlier. Then you were told which doctor to see, and that doctor only gave you a few minutes. During that short appointment, everything felt disorganized, and you really didn't understand what was happening. You certainly knew nothing about the costs.

That doctor sent you for more blood work and an MRI, just like those you had a few months earlier. You felt that was both a waste of time and money.

You are glad that your fellow Americans chose the free market to deliver health care services, unlike your Canadian cousin who has been waiting to see the specialist for two months.

So, what is holding us back from moving ahead to implement this new and exciting health care system?

CHAPTER 24
UNLEASHING A CURE FOR WHAT AILS U.S. HEALTH CARE

Reining in the high costs of health care while increasing quality and quantity is not so complicated. It starts with choosing to say "no" to a government monopoly, and "yes" to free market competition.

Our current health care system, in many ways, resembles the AT&T monopoly before the break up. Federal and state governments, through Medicare and Medicaid, plus scores of other tax-funded programs, pay 46 percent of the nation's health care bills while serving 26 percent of the population. Through this large share of the market, governments already exert immense control over the delivery of health care.

In addition, politicians have micromanaged private health care by placing increasing demands on providers and payers. Their actions have added tens of billions of dollars in cost each year.

Meanwhile, most people have been shielded from the real cost of health care. They have paid a monthly premium, low or no deductibles, and small office and prescription drug co-pays, but never know the actual cost.

Doctors, hospitals, and clinics have adapted their practices to suit the payers – Medicare, Medicaid, HMOs and insurance companies – not the patient. It is wrong to assume that providers and payers like it this way. They know that everyone would benefit if patients, instead of politicians, were in control, and competitive forces shaped the market, as with telephone and long distance service.

The cure for U.S. health care requires breaking the government monopoly and letting a truly free market determine costs and develop efficiencies through competition. The success of such a system depends on you being able to function as a consumer, purchasing health care in the same manner as you do with nearly every other product, service or device.

Injecting competition and information into your purchasing decision would make an immense difference in the cost, quality and supply of health care services and how providers deliver them. Lasik surgery, heart scans, and Loradatine instead of Claritin, have shown us this tremendous potential.

CURING HEALTH CARE

Earlier in this book we talked about three major players in health care: patients, providers, and payers. We have discussed, as well, the central role already played by governments in determining and controlling the health care economy. All health care reform requires each of these players to take the cure.

The entire health care system must purposefully push ahead adapting electronic technology to streamline the entire process. As shown in our office call of the future, getting this right is one of the more important requirements of reducing cost, while increasing quality. Patients, payers, and providers must be linked together with a seamless system of record-keeping and bill paying. This will reduce wasted time, do away with unnecessary diagnostic tests, and ensure that money is spent more wisely. Providers will be paid more efficiently, and their record-keeping requirements greatly reduced.

The cost of creating this electronic integration is a fraction of the savings it will create year after year. You will receive higher quality care at reduced cost. It might even save your life, given the increased speed, quality, and quantity of information available to medical providers.

CURING GOVERNMENT HEALTH CARE

Since the federal government and each state government has become so entangled in our health care system, we must start our reform effort with them. While it is doing so, it must quit mandating new requirements onto the rest of us.

The government must provide us with a clear, honest appraisal of its health care and administrative costs.

Medicare must be addressed seriously. The United States cannot afford to shackle young working couples with the burden of providing health care services to 77 million baby boomers. Bearing that cost is unfair. This subject is complex, and our next book will directly address it. There is, however, no time to waste. We urge Congress to get going on this, to correct the structural problems that allow Americans with large estates to have their health care bills paid by working people who are struggling to build their own financial security. That is just plain wrong.

Governments must work to privatize as much of its health care system as possible. Where this is not feasible, all government health care programs should be coordinated in such a way as to eliminate massive waste from overlapping programs.

Governments should quit subsidizing health care and health insurance for those who can, and should, buy their own. It makes no sense for families earning $50,000 or $75,000 a year, or more, to receive health care through government programs or paid for by subsidized insurance premiums.

Writing the eligibility rules for taxpayer-subsidized health care programs must be taken away from government officials. These decisions must be made by non-government officials who have no vested interest in growing the number of people that use government programs.

Community health centers, charitable health care, and some level of government-paid health insurance should continue to provide high-quality services for those who are truly poor.

In America, people are free to choose to purchase health insurance or not. It is their right. It would be wrong for governments to mandate that everyone must own health insurance. Besides, it will fail in its mission to reduce the uninsured rate to zero. The only thing it will accomplish is to increase administrative cost to police and enforce insurance laws for our mobile American society.

We must recognize that a sizable number of us refuse to see medical doctors, and instead, trust in treatments that will never be covered by insurance. It is wrong to force them to buy something they will never use.

We see no reason that government employee health benefits should cost more than those of private employees. Governments must adopt health benefit plans more in line with those of private industry.

Governments should quit trying to micromanage private health care, but instead, perform their constitutional duties. Wrongdoers should be vigorously prosecuted and punished. Monopolies should be broken, to encourage competition. Patents must be carefully issued and aggressively protected, but once they have expired, governments should do nothing to inhibit the free market from developing them into new, competitive drugs, medical devices and services.

The Food and Drug Administration should continue to review and approve new drugs and medical devices to ensure their safety, and it should continue to enforce safety standards. However, the FDA must do all it can to reduce wasted and unnecessary time and expense that serves only to drive up the cost of medical advances, and it must continuously streamline its processes.

Governments should remove themselves from the process of deciding which benefits should be covered by non-government insurance plans. The decision about which benefits to offer in non-government plans should be left up to insurance companies and those who purchase insurance. Free market forces will shape health insurance policies that people will want to buy, that they can afford, and that provide the benefits most important to them.

Governments should change tax policy so that all health expenses are fully tax deductible.

Governments should do nothing to inhibit the growth or use of health savings accounts.

Congress should pass legislation that prohibits any government from trying to influence the number of doctors entering practice, as congress intended to do with H.R. 3600 in 1994. Medical schools are perfectly capable and better suited to determine where to focus their training programs than any government planner ever could be.

State governments must change medical malpractice tort law to protect against unreasonable and expensive lawsuits. This must be done so as to ensure that wrongdoers are severely punished, but recognize that sometimes, mistakes are made. When people suffer as a result of the malicious intent of a provider, that doctor should be locked up, and the patient should receive reasonable payment for real losses. When mistakes are made that result in suffering and death, reasonable payment should be made. Punitive damages, however, designed to punish providers and enrich lawyers must be either capped at a specific dollar amount, or those proceeds must be paid to the state, not to lawyers and plaintiffs. And if the states refuse to make these reforms, then, and only then, should the federal government pass national legislation to provide these protections.

CURING THE PAYERS

The health insurance industry is remarkably adaptable to market forces. Once it is freed from massive government influence, it can create new, competitive, and affordable insurance products custom-designed to meet the needs of large groups, small groups, and individuals.

We believe that the market will force health insurers to devise new, affordable catastrophic health insurance plans. Among the most exciting of these are Health Savings Accounts (HSAs).

An HSA would serve at least three purposes. You would be able to set aside tax-free funds to pay your first dollar medical expenses. Those HSA funds, if not used, can be accumulated and applied to future health care expenses, or as part of retirement savings, and even passed on to heirs. Most importantly, however, is that you would actually see and pay for many of your health care costs from your HSA. That will help you be more careful how those dollars are spent, making you a better health care consumer.

Insurance companies should make health care pricing transparent. This means it would be easy for you to retrieve the price of a health care service from all the providers in your area. Before you ever receive a service, or purchase a drug or device, you will know how much your insurance will pay. This information will be available by phone, internet, or online chats; in any form that is easy to retrieve and understand.

Insurance companies will become involved in helping you assess your health, and joining with you and your doctor in setting wellness goals. They will make available medical encyclopedias with information about diseases, nutrition, surgeries, systems, tests, and other special topics, all available for instant access via the internet. They will provide self-help guides to understand common, chronic illnesses like asthma, diabetes, and high blood pressure. This is just the beginning.

We believe that, freed from government mandates, innovative cutting-edge insurance companies will emerge. That is what will happen as creative entrepreneurs are unshackled from government mandates to create innovative insurance products and services for millions of willing buyers.

CURING THE PROVIDERS

The key to making a free market health care system work is information.

Patients must be able to see the prices charged for care before making a decision about whether to use services, forgo a procedure, or go to a different provider. We know this is a daunting task, especially for hospitals, but it needs to be done. If auto makers, telephone companies, and Lasik surgeons can do this, so can they.

Doctors must know the costs of diagnostic tests before sending patients to a lab or clinic. They must partner with their patients to make sure that each test is necessary and provides good value.

Doctors must recognize that patients are fully capable, working in partnership with them and their insurance companies, to make wise spending choices. To do so, they need information.

Governments, payers, and providers agree: Health care pricing has become so complex that even they do not understand it. The government has used the issue of complexity to position itself to define what comprises a necessary procedure. Insurance companies have used it to attempt to impose quality and efficiency controls on providers. Doctors say that the billing process is too complicated. Hospitals just refuse to disclose their charges. The patient is left at the mercy of this complexity. That must change. The consumer must be able to access the price of health care in the same way that they can pre-determine the price of any other product or service.

The patient-doctor relationship will be enriched as patients are empowered to help themselves. Providers must be able to present easily understood information to patients about their health care needs, and make it clear to patients that they are responsible to use it.

As hard as it may be for independent-minded doctors, their professional associations must develop science-based practice guidelines by which they guide their medical practice. Besides providing healthier patient outcomes and reducing waste in health care spending, it would also insulate doctors and hospitals from nuisance malpractice lawsuits. Governments should not play any role in the development or implementing of practice guidelines. These should be the product of professional medical associations and health care scholars acting through free associations. We believe that letting the government help develop practice guidelines would open the door to rationing health care for those most in need – the elderly and those with chronic illnesses.

Providers, especially doctors, must make the patient a partner in deciding on health care strategies. Medical practice must be patient-focused, in the same way that retailers focus on pleasing customers. Since patients will be armed with information about their medical conditions and expected to act on it, and they will know costs and authorize payment of the bills, doctors will naturally develop a close relationship with them. Remember, if the patient is unhappy with the doctor's service, they will not authorize payment.

As doctors develop practice teams, they will be freed up to spend more time with each patient, and ensure that they understand and agree with what is being done.

CURING PATIENTS

What is your part in health care reform? It starts with changing your mind and your habits about how to access and pay for health care. It means moving from the entitlement mentality to one of empowerment, knowing and believing that you are fully capable of managing your personal health, and making good financial decisions. We are very upbeat about this.

None of the above-mentioned reforms will work well unless you are activated to fully participate in your own health care decisions. When a doctor presents you with facts, references, and understandable and easily available materials, you must follow through and do your part. Your medical outcomes will be far more successful when you and your doctor agree on, and are committed to the same health care strategy.

Health care professionals across the world agree on this one thing: that all of us need to take better care of our bodies. We need to exercise, watch our diet, and guard against dangerous, risky behaviors. For as Pogo said to Porky, "Yep, son, we have met the enemy and he is us."[1]

---

1. Walt Kelly, *Pogo: We Have Met the Enemy and He Is Us*, 1972.

CHAPTER 25
MAKING YOUR CHOICE
BECAUSE YOUR HEALTH MATTERS

Early in this book we described four major forces that contributed to the great success of the United States' economy, and our health care system. Those major forces were a culture of work, private ownership and capitalism, discretionary income, and technological advances.

America flourished because we cherish freedom, and honored the sacred nature of human life. Phase I in the health care socialization process, however, has begun to move us away from what made us great. Phase I is marked by these signs:

> The costs of health care services are unknown to its users, so services are perceived to be free or almost free.

> People believe that health care is an inalienable right like life, liberty, and the pursuit of happiness.

> Since health care is a right, everyone is entitled to it.

> Everyone is entitled to have others help

pay for their health care, even if they refuse to insure themselves.

These Phase I characteristics are at odds with the values upon which we have built our nation and economy. They have made us dependent on others to take care of our health care needs.

Today, a powerful coalition of political, cultural, business, and religious leaders believe we should go the rest of the way and adopt a national health care plan. They call it universal health care, mandatory health insurance, or a single-payer system. They would have us enter Phase II of the socialization process.

Before we decide to move to Phase II, we need to consider these chilling words about the National Health Service of the United Kingdom: "The [NHS] ministry that provides guidance on public health issues in Great Britain is proposing to *deny treatment to patients based on age.* That's the ultimate end for universal health care."[1] [Emphasis added]

The NHS' proposal is a rational one for a health care system limited by a global budget. Health care must be cost-effective. The system will fund as much as it can afford, and what it can afford will be determined by that which is perceived to benefit the most people. Caring for ailing senior citizens, those with lifetime chronic illness, and tiny premature babies, is not cost-effective. It is hard to imagine an America in which these vulnerable people are allowed to suffer and die just because we refuse to spend what it takes to care for them. Yet, that is the logical outcome of entering Phase II, and embracing a national health care system.

---

1. "Forget It, Grandma: Universal Health Care Means Rationing Treatment," *Investor's Business Daily*, May 6, 2005, http://www.investors.com/editorial/issues01.asp?v=5/6

"Health care is either going to be allocated by prices or by government, which in the latter case means price controls and waiting lines."[2] Is that what you want?

A CHANGE IN NATIONAL CHARACTER

Americans have always understood the idea of self-sacrifice. It is why we continue to send our soldiers to war, why we fight to preserve freedom and liberty. Our current health care system still maintains vestiges of these ideas, but if we move to Phase II of the socialization of health care, it will mean we have abandoned our core values.

By choosing Phase II, we will be telling the government that we are no longer interested in personal responsibility. We will be saying that freedom and liberty are less important than having someone else care for us, even though we know that they, not us, will make the rules. If we choose Phase II, we will do it knowing that others will lose out, even while we are left to enjoy our own lives.

At our nation's founding we embraced the principle that the greatest demonstration of love is the willingness to lay down one's life for another. Though we are seldom called upon to make the ultimate sacrifice, we are often called upon to sacrifice some of our assets to provide care to our loved ones, and to care for ourselves. The socialist sees these issues differently.

The socialist practices the idea that the greatest good comes when the government distributes benefits based on the fairness principle. For this to happen, we must all agree that everyone is entitled to benefit from the sweat of someone else's brow. Then we will hand those responsibilities to the government. In a socialist system, however, we soon

---

2. "The Health Care Opportunity," *The Wall Street Journal*, Feb. 2, 2006, A14.

learn that the strong survive and the weakest must be allowed to die.

Let's be frank. Compassion costs money. Freedom costs money. Governments do not offer compassion, they just distribute benefits. To access those benefits, we must sacrifice freedom. We replace freedom with rigid protocols and global budgets.

Why would you want to embrace what continues to fail elsewhere? You would only do so if you were uninformed, and felt hopeless and defeated, as though there is nothing you can personally do to control cost. Maybe your sense of compassion causes you to believe that the uninsured are being denied health care. To include them, you might have concluded, requires government takeover of everyone's health care. But to believe this is to believe a myth. To believe this means that we see no other options.

Choosing Phase II will be done if you believe the myth that an American socialized system will be different from those of other countries; that somehow, Americans can do socialism better than they can. It will not be long before artificial knees, hips, and motorized carts are replaced by canes and walkers, devices far more cost-effective than surgery.

Moving to Phase II of the socialization process will be a clear sign that, as a people, we have lost an essential aspect of our American way of life: our desire to govern our own lives. Giving up has never been part of the American vocabulary.

Why would you want to give up on yourself when there is such a better alternative? Why would you and your fellow Americans, living in the world's wealthiest nation, want to entrust your life to government planners?

REFORM MUST HAPPEN,
BUT OUR CHOICE OF REFORM IS CRUCIAL

We never set out to write a definitive book on how to reform U.S. health care. In chapter 24 we laid out guidelines, but the details are best worked out by those with the financial, scientific, and academic resources it requires. What is certain is that health care reform must happen.

The key to successful reform is engaging you and all health care consumers in spending decisions, and in partnering with doctors on a personal health strategy. We have absolute confidence that you are up to this task, that you are fully capable of managing your own life.

America's first settlers at Jamestown faced a similarly tough decision in 1612. They chose the right road; it required everyone to work and provide for their own needs. They, and other early Americans, would be shocked that today we are so dependent on others to protect our lives and fortunes. They would see how Americans have been gradually duped into believing that they are entitled to benefit at someone else's expense.

At Jamestown, the entitlement mentality road had led to suffering, starvation, and death. Then, they chose the road that led to free markets, private ownership, personal responsibility, and hard work. They decided against the entitlement mentality. Four hundred years later, we still benefit from their decision.

You do not need the government to manage your life. You have the ability to tell the free market what you will accept, and how much you will pay. No one can do this better than you, because frankly, your health matters more to you than anyone else.

BIBLIOGRAPHY
With page numbers where each cite is used.

ARTICLES

"A Primer on Health Care, Health Care Puzzles," Tomoko Furukawa, *The JapanTimes Online,* Nov. 2004: 172, 226.

"American Medical Association Patient Care Physician Survey, 2001:" 191.

"Americans Living Longer, Experts cite better treatments for heart disease," *HealthScoutNews Reporter,* Mar. 14, 2003: 6.

"Analysts suggest mandatory health coverage," Andrew Damstedt, *The Washington Times,* May 5, 2005: 183, 184.

"Are the Uninsured Freeloaders?" National Center for Policy Analysis, Brief Analysis No. 120, Aug. 10, 1994: 178.

"Bulletin of the World Health Organization," March 2004: 239, 242, 243.

"Census Bureau's Uninsured Number Indicates Third Increase in a Row," FamiliesUSA.org, Aug. 26, 2004: 177.

"Characteristics of the Nonelderly with Selected Sources of Health Insurance and Lengths of Uninsured Spells," Craig Copeland, EBRI Issue Brief No. 198, June 1998, Employee Benefit Research Institute, Washington, D.C.: 180.

"Congressman's Report," Honorable Morris Udahl, D-Arizona, March 31, 1965: 111.

"Defusing the Medicare Time Bomb," Robert E. Moffit, Ph.D. and Andrew Grossman, The Heritage Foundation, May 26, 2005: 126.

"Derm Career," American Board of Dermatology, 2005: 60.

"Expensive Drugs Drive Up Health Care Costs," Millie Munshi, Associated Press, Washingtonpost.com, June 13, 2005: 150.

"Experts Sound Medicare Alarm: Observers say the program will be in more trouble than Social Security," Bennett Roth, *Houston Chronicle,* Feb. 6, 2005: 118.

"For Some A Painful Cut," Warren Wolfe, *Minneapolis Star-Tribune,* Jan. 31, 2005: 133.

"For Young Doctors, It's Not Marcus Welby's Practice," Richard L. Reece, 2005: 11, 66, 67.

"Forget It, Grandma: Universal Health Care Means Rationing Treatment," *Investor's Business Daily,* May 6, 2005: 312.

"Free trade tack for drug imports," John Goodman, *The Washington Times,* Jan. 31, 2005: 141.

"Fundamentals of the Prescription Drug Market," Christine Provost Peters, NHPF Background Paper, Aug. 24, 2004: 142, 146, 147, 151, 152, 153, 154.

"Generic Drug Prices, a Canada-US Comparison," Palmer D'Angelo Consulting Inc., Aug. 2002: 141, 142.

"German Health Care System in Transition, The difficult way to balance Cost Containment and Solidarity," Prof. Dr. J. Matthias Graf von der Schulenburg, *European Journal of Health Economics*, 2005: 248, 249, 252, 254, 256, 257, 258.

"GM's UAW Retirees Face Health Care Costs, Deal Would End Free Coverage," Amy Joyce, *The Washington Post*, Oct. 21, 2005: 105.

"Health and Health Care of Japanese-American Elders," Marianne K.G. Tannabe, M.D., Stanford University, 2005: 171.

"Health Care Cost, HMOs, PPOs, EPOs:" 90.

"Health Care in a Free Society, Rebutting the Myths of National Health Insurance," John C. Goodman, National Center for Policy Analysis, Dallas, TX, Jan. 27, 2005: 202, 209, 211, 212, 218, 222, 224.

"Health Care Puzzles," Tomoko Furukawa, *The Japan Times Online*, Nov. 16, 2004: 226, 228.

"Health care reforms in Europe and their implications for Japan," Peter C. Smith, *The Japanese Journal of Social Security Policy: Vol. 3, No. 2*, Dec. 2004: 225, 259, 260, 261.

"Health Care Spending in the United States Slows for the First Time in Seven Years," *CMS News*, Centers for Medicare and Medicaid Services, Jan. 11, 2005: 117, 127, 135.

"Health Costs Absorb One-Quarter of Economic Growth, 2000-2005," Alan Sager and Deborah Socolar, Boston University: 81.

"History of Health Insurance Benefits," Facts from EBRI, March 2002: 85.

"How Health Care Costs Are Transforming Health Benefits," Theodore Loftness, M.D., Slide 18, Medica Broker Forum, Sept. 14, 2005: 153.

"How to Stack the Deck in Your Favor," Glenn R. Stout, M.D., Senior

FAA Medical Examiner: 54, 55.

"Illegals: The Real Cause of Health Insurance Crisis," Jim Meyers, NewsMax.com, May 2, 2005: 183.

"IMS Reports 8.3 Percent Dollar Growth in 2004 U.S. Prescription Sales," Feb. 14, 2005: 137.

"International pricing and distribution of therapeutic pharmaceuticals: an ethical minefield," Joan Buckley and Seamus OL Tuama, *Business Ethics, A European Review, Vol. 14, No. 5*, April 2005: 147, 151.

"Interview With Newt Gingrich," *Limbaugh Letter*, August, 2005: 118.

"Labour Market and Social Policy, Occasional Papers No 56: An Assessment of the Performance of the Japanese Health Care System," Directorate for Education, Employment, Labour, and Social Affairs Committee, OECD, Dec. 2001: 226, 227, 228, 229, 230, 231, 232, 233.

"Look to Japan on Health," Nadeem Esmail, *Fraser Forum*, Nov. 2004: 231, 232.

"Medical Malpractice Insurance," Insurance Information Institute, June, 2003: 80, 81.

"Medical miscalculation creates doctor shortage. After a glut was predicted a decade ago, the number of physicians isn't keeping up with the demands of a wealthy, aging population," Dennis Cauchon, *USA TODAY*, 3/3/2005: 68.

MetLife General News: Press release, April 2002: 22 MinnesotaCare Premium Table, July 2005-June 2006, 4. 133.

"Minnesota Health Care Marketplace Reform," William Wenmark, 2005: 92.

"Minor Oxygen Deprivation at Birth Can Dull Mental Skills, Threshold for damage is lower than previously believed, study finds," Jennifer Thomas, *HealthScoutNews Reporter*: 162.

"Nation's Largest Health Coalition Calls For Sweeping Changes in Health Care System," National Health Care Coalition, July 20, 2005: 179.

"Pharmaceutical Marketing, Time for a Change," Joan Buckley, *The Electronic Journal of Business and Organizational Studies, Vol. 9, No. 2*: 152.

"Premature Babies: Study: 'Miracle babies' have disabilities at age 6, A study in Britain found nearly half of all extremely premature babies had significant disabilities by age 6. Some doubted the study applied to U.S. practices today," Stephanie Nano, Associated Press Writer: 160, 161.

"Reform of Germany's Health Care Market," Prof. Dr. Stefan Felder, Institute of Social Medicine and Health Economics, University of Magdeburg, Germany, Maritim ProArte Hotel, Berlin, revised version July 4, 2002: 257.

"Remember Cost Control," Peter Peterson, *Newsweek,* July 25, 1994, as quoted in the *"Cato Institute Tax and Budget Bulletin*, Sept. 2003: 117.

"Santé to the French health system," Patrick Lenain, Economics department, October 2000: 237, 238, 240, 244.

"State/Local Government Pay & Benefits Much Higher Than in Private Sector, But Jobs, Skills Differ," Employee Benefit Research Institute, April 6, 2005: 270.

"Summary Report, 2005 Review of Physician Recruitment Incentives," Merritt, Hawkins & Associates: 65.

"The French Health Care System: A Brief Overview," Presentation prepared for the Permanent Working Group of European Junior Doctors, October 2001: 240, 241, 243, 240.

"The German Health Care System at the Crossroads," Prof. Dr. J. Mathias Graf von der Schulenberg, *Health Economics, Vol. 3,* 1994: 255.

"The Health Care Opportunity," *The Wall Street Journal,* Feb. 2, 2006: 313.

"The Private Cost of Public Queues," Nadeem Esmail, Fraser Institute, March 2005: 211.

"Tort Reform," *News Batch*, February, 2005: 75, 77, 78.

"U.S. Infant Mortality Rate Rises for First time Since 1958, CDC Report Finds," Across the Nation, *California Health Line*, Feb. 12, 2004: 163.

"U.S. Tort Costs: 2003 Update, Trends and Findings on the Costs of the U.S. Tort System," Tillinghast Towers-Perrin: 75.

"What Health Insurance Crisis?".David Gratzer, *The Los Angeles Times*, Aug. 29, 2004: 183

"Who Should Pay for What," Erica Seiguer, Harvard Medical School, 2003: 161.

"2004 Survey of Physicians 50 to 65 Years Old, Based on 2003 Data," Merritt, Hawkins & Associates: 63, 67, 69.

BOOKS & BOOKLETS

An Introduction to the Study of Labor Problems, Gordon S. Watkins, Thomas Crowell Company, 1922: 201.

Bulletin of the World Health Organization, March, 2004, 82(3), page 232. 25.

Concise Encyclopedia of Economics: 13.

Freakonomics, Steven D. Levitt and Stephen J. Dubner, William Morrow, 2005: 177.

Health Care Systems in Transition, Reinhard Busse and Annette Riesberg, World Health Organization, 2004: 22. 250, 252.

Health Forum, Annual Survey, *(1990-2003),* American Hospital Association: 191.

Lessons Learned From Other Health Care Systems, Prof. Dr. Klaus-Dirk Henke, Prof. Robert F. Rich, Prof. Dr. Hilmar Stolte, M.D., Technische Universitat Berlin, Nov. 2004: 254, 256.

Medicaid At-a-Glance, 2005; A Medicaid Information Source, Centers for Medicare and Medicaid Services: 129, 132, 134.

Medicaid At-a-Glance, 2003, A Medicaid Information Source, Centers for Medicare and Medicaid Services: 124.

Pogo: We Have Met the Enemy and He Is Us, Walt Kelly, 1972: 310.

"Soviet Ownership," *Great Soviet Encyclopedia,* 1975: 200.

The 2002 Employer Benefits Study, U.S. Chamber of Commerce, 2002: 105.

The Artful Askers Workbook, Bob Vickers, National Heritage Foundation, February, 2005: 11. 37.

The Uninsured in America, Blue Cross, Blue Shield Foundation, 2005: 180, 181, 182.

To Change the Heart of Man, Dave Racer, 2006: 43, 48.

Voices of Health Care Reform, Practice Support Resources, Inc., Richard L. Reece, M.D., 2005: 59, 61, 266.

EMAILS

DFCRCOMM (HRSA), April 19, 2005, in an email to Mr. Racer, responding to his question: 191.

Email received on May 13, 2005, from DOT-DMV Traf-Acc-Sec: (traf-acc-sec.dmv@dot.state.wi.us): 187.

Heart Institute of the Cascades, for 2005, via email to the author on 11/21/05: 74, 289.

Mr. James Genetti, Idaho Department of Transportation email: 187.

Peter, Ashkenaz, Deputy Director, CMS Media, Centers for Medicare and Medicaid, via email, Feb. 13, 2006: 125.

INFORMATION RECEIVED FROM WWW.INFOPLEASE.COM

"Area and Population of Countries, Mid-2005 Estimates:" 204.

"Crime Rates for Selected Large Cities, 2002 (offenses known to the police per 100,000 inhabitants):" 157.

"Crude Birth and Death Rates for Selected Countries (per 1,000 population):" 170, 239.

"Economic Statistics by Country, 2004:" 204.

"Infant Mortality and Life Expectancy for Selected Countries, 2004:" 173.

"Definition of Free Enterprise:" 201.

"Median Income of Households by Selected Characteristics, 2004:" 112.

LAWS OR BILLS

H.R. 3600, 103rd Congress, 1994: 52, 69, 79, 123, 272, 273, 274, 275, 276.

MN Statutes, 62E04, 62E06: 134.

TABLES AND DATA SOURCES

Average Length of Stay by Diagnostic Category, 2003, QuickStats, U.S. Centers for Disease Control: 232.

Basic Structural Statistics, for 2003, Main Economic Indicators, 2005, OECD: 228.

Employment, Hours, and Earnings from the Current Employment Statistics Survey, U.S. Bureau of Labor Statistics, Dept of Labor, US Gov't.: 135.

FY 2005 Budget in Brief, Health Resources and Services Administration, United States: 192, 193.

Health Spending and Resources, OECD in Figures, 2005 edition: 233.

Infant Mortality and Life Expectancy for Selected Countries, 2004, U.S. Census Bureau, International Data Base: 227.

Minnesota Rate Sheet, 2005, Blue Cross, Blue Shield: 133.

National Health Expenditures Accounts: Definitions, Sources, and Methods Used in the NHEA 2004, Centers for Medicare and Medicaid: 268, 269.

National Health Expenditures by Type of Service & Source of Funds: Calendar Years 1960-2004, Centers for Medicaid & Medicare, U.S. Government: 51, 86, 88.

National Vital Statistics Report, Vol 50, No 12, U.S. Census Bureau, Aug. 28, 2002: 19, 158, 161, 163, 164.

No. 114. National Health Expenditures–Summary, 1960-2002, and Projections, 2003-2013, Abstract of the United States, Bureau of the Census: 88.

Organization for Economic Co-Operation and Development (OECD) Life Expectancy Tables, June 2005: 227.

Organization for Economic Co-Operation and Development (OECD), Life Expectancy Table for 2003: 167.

Social Security & Medicare Tax Rates, Updated December 23, 2002, U.S. Social Security Administration: 113.

Table 010. Infant Mort Rates & Life Exp at Birth, by Sex, U.S. Census Bureau International Data Base: 21, 159.

Table 1: National Health Expenditures Aggregate and Per Capita Amounts, and Average Annual Percent Growth, by Source of Funds, Selected Calendar Years: 1980-2003, CMS, Health and Human Services, United States: 33, 51, 52, 83, 101, 202.

Table 3: National Health Expenditures, by Source of Funds and Type of Expenditure: Selected Calendar Years 1998-2003, Centers for Medicare and Medicaid: 268, 269.

Table 4: Personal Health Care Expenditures Aggregate and Per Capita Amounts and Distribution, by Source of Funds: Selected Calendar Years 1980-2003, Centers for Medicare and Medicaid Services, U.S. Government: 128.

Table 12: Per Enrollee Expenditures and Growth in Medicare Spending and Private Health Insurance Premiums, Calendar Years 1969-2003, Centers for Medicare and Medicaid Services, United States: 89, 97, 110, 113, 121, 267.

Table HI-1. Health Insurance Coverage Status and Type of Coverage by Sex, Race and Hispanic Origin: 1987 to 2004,"CMS, Health and Human Services, United States: 33, 37, 84, 267.

Table No. 139, Statistical abstract of the United States, 2003, Bureau of the Census: 101.

Table No. 13, Statistical abstract of the United States, 2000-2004: 170.

Total expenditure on health–% of gross domestic product, OECD, 2003: 25, 204.

WEBSITES

"About Health Care, About Missions, Values, Activities:" http://www.hc-sc.gc/ahc-asc/activit/aboutapropros/index_e.html, 208.

"About Health Centers, History of Community Health Centers," National Association of Community Health Centers: http://www.nache.com/about/about-centers.asp. 191, 192, 193.

"About WHO:" http://www.who.int/about/en/, 237.

"Consumer Price Index, 1913-,"
Minneapolis Fed Reserve Bank:
http://www.minneapolisfed.org/
Research/data/us/calc/
hist1913.cfm, 97.

"Coverage Center Page," Centers for
Medicare and Medicaid Services,
United States:
http://www.cms.hhs.gov/center/
coverage.asp., 110.

"Fast Facts on U.S. Hospitals from
AHA Hospital Statistics, 2006:"
http://www.aha.org/aha/resource_cen
ter/fastfacts/fast_facts_US_hospi-
tals.html 44

"Insure Kids Now:"
http://www.insurekidsnow.gov/, 189.

"Physician Compensation Salary
Survey, in Practice Three Plus
Years," June 30, 2005:
http://www.physicianssearch.com/
physician/salary2.html, June 30,
2005, 65.

"Prepaid Health Care Act:"
http://www.hawaii.gov/labor/ded/
aboutphc.shtml, 188.

"President's Advisory Commission
on Consumer Protection and Quality
in the Health Care Industry:"
http://www.hcqualitycommission.gov
/charter.html, 102, 103, 104.

"The Free Dictionary," by Farlex:
http://financialdictionary.thefreedic-
tionary.com/Free+Market, 281.

"The History of Penicillin," Mary
Bellis:
http://inventors.about.com/library
/inventors/blpenicillin.htm, 48.

"A Litigation Digest & Directory:"
http://www.morelaw.com/verdicts/
43, 78.

"Ads, Promotions Drive Up Drug
Costs, Drugmakers Spend Billions
Reaching Consumers, Docs," Patricia Barry, March 2002:
http://www.aarp.org, 153.

"At LasikPlus Vision Centers, All
We Do is Perform Laser Vision Correction:" http://www.lasikplus.com/,
288.

"Choice for patients who have waited six months:"
http://www.dh.uk/PolicyAndGuid-
ance/PatientChoice/Choice/
ChoiceArticle/fs/, 223.

"Cost of Lasik and other corrective
eye surgery," Liz Segre:
http://www.allaboutvision.com/
visionsurgery/cost.htm, 287.

"Healthcare System:" Japan Pharmaceutical Manufacturers Association,
http://www.jpma.or.jp/12english/
guide_industry/healthcare/
healthcare.html, 226.

"History of Lasik Surgery," Philip
Colenda, MD, PC, FAAO:
http://www.westchestervision.com/hi
storyoflasik.html. 287

"Leading expert calls for NHS to
tackle soaring levels of workforce
stress," June 17, 2005:
http://www.nhsconfed.org/press/
releases/workforce_stress.asp, 220.

"Performance Indicators for Acute
and Specialist Trust:"
http://nhs.uk/England/About-
TheNhs/StarRatings/
AcuteSpecialPI.cmsx, 4. 218.

"September 18, 2005 Bundestag
Election Final Results – Federal
Republic of Germany Totals," Election Resources on the Internet: Elections to the German Bundestag:
http://electionresources.org/de/, 253.

"Terminating stagnation – redesigning the system," German Association
of Research-Based Pharmaceutical
Companies, 2005:
http://www.vfa.de/en/articles/
art_2002-02_001.html, 255.

"The NHS from 1948-1957:"
http://www.nhs.uk/England/About-
TheNhsHistory/1948-1957.cmsx,
205, 273.

"Top All-Time Donor Profiles:"
http://www.opensecrets.org/, 79.

Bureau of Primary Health Care:
http://bphc.hrsa.gov/programs/CHC
Programinfo.asp, 191.

Inflation Calculator, U.S. Census
Bureau: http://data.bls.gov/
cgi-bin/cpicalc.pl, 284.

Maternal and Child Health Bureau:
http://www.hrsa.gov/annualreport/
part5.htm, 194.

Social Security Reform Center:
http://www.socialsecurityreform.org/
problems/index.cfm, 118.

U.S./Canadian Price Comparisons,
Oct. 2004:
http://www.fda.gov/oc/opacom/hot-
topics/importdrugs/CanadaRX.html,
141.

http://www.CanadaDrugs.com, June
23, 2005, 140.

http://www.walgreens.com, June 23,
2005, 140.

Wikipedia, the free encyclopedia
online, 160.

http://www.nhs.uk/England/About-
The Nhs/History/1948-1957.cmsx
215, 216, 220.

http://www.nhs.uk/England/
AboutTheNhs/History/
Before1948.cmsx, 216.

http://www.nhs.uk?England/About-
TheNhs/History/1978-1987.cmsx,
221.

OTHER DOCUMENTS USED
FOR BACKGROUND OR
ADDITIONAL CONSIDERATION

"Conn. Enacts Law on Infertility
Treatment," Susan Haigh, *The Hart-
ford Courant*, Sep. 6, 1005.

"French Sesam Vitale Health Card,"
Smart Card Alliance, 2005.

"Goals that Keep the Promise of the
'H'...," American Hospital Association.

Health – The German Way,
(Excerpted), Hyde Flippo, Passport
Books, 1997.

"Health Care: Making the Best of a
Bad Bargain," Michael Hatch, Atty.
Gen., State of MN, 2005.

"LISTENING TO MINNESOTANS:
TRANSFORMING MINNESOTA'S
HEALTH CARE SYSTEM," Report
of the Minnesota Citizens Forum on
Health Care Costs Feb. 23, 2004.

"Physicians' Plan for a Healthy Min-
nesota: The MMA's Proposal for
Health Care Reform," Minnesota
Medical Assn., 2005.

"PROVIDING COVERAGE TO
ALL: MMA'S WHITE PAPER ON
HEALTH CARE REFORM IN
MAINE," Maine Medical Assn.,
May 1, 2003.

"Spending Pressures Continue
Despite Revenue Growth," National
Governors' Assn., 2005.

"TEXAS MEDICAL ASSOCIA-
TION'S HEALTHY VISION,"
TMA, 2005.

"The State and Pattern of HEALTH
Information Technology Adoption,"
Kateryna Fonkych & Roger Taylor,
Rand Corp., 2005.

"Toward Sustainable Health Care
Systems: Strategies in Health Insur-
ance Schemes in Germany, Japan,
and the Netherlands," Klaus-Dirk
Henke and Jonas Schreyögg, Berlin,
May 2004."